Coma and Disorders of Consciousness

Caroline Schnakers • Steven Laureys
Editors

Coma and Disorders of Consciousness

Springer

Editors
Caroline Schnakers, Ph.D.
Coma Science Group
Cyclotron Research Center
University of Liège, Liège
Belgium

Steven Laureys, M.D., Ph.D.
Coma Science Group
Cyclotron Research Center
University of Liège, Liège
Belgium

ISBN 978-1-4471-2439-9 ISBN 978-1-4471-2440-5 (eBook)
DOI 10.1007/978-1-4471-2440-5
Springer Dordrecht Heidelberg New York London

Library of Congress Control Number: 2012940279

Printed on acid-free paper

Springer is part of Springer Science+Business Media (www.springer.com)

To medical teams and families we see every day and who inspire us.

Foreword I

Consciousness is synonymous with human existence. Rene Descarte's bold proclamation, "Cogito ergo sum" (I think therefore I am), elegantly captures this premise. The clear inference here is that self-doubt about one's own existence establishes proof of one's existence. We exist because we know we exist. But how does one come to know that someone else is aware of his existence? Without direct access to knowledge of the self, it is impossible to prove (or disprove) the awareness of another. In normal consciousness, this problem is obviated by the multitude of behavioral expressions of conscious awareness manifested by living beings nearly every waking moment. Words, gestures and actions, the "stuff" of consciousness, provide compelling evidence of the inner life of another.

A small but significant percentage (5–10%) of those who sustain severe acquired brain injury experience prolonged disturbance in consciousness. Most will eventually recover at least basic capacity for self and environmental awareness, but this may not occur for many months and, in some cases, years. During this period of severely altered consciousness, one's existence may be stripped of the usual harbingers of an active inner life. Sensory, motor, language, perceptual and drive systems may all be compromised in the aftermath of severe brain injury. Consequently, the repertoire of behaviors available to signal retention of conscious awareness may be dramatically narrowed or lost altogether. This predicament presents one of humankind's greatest existential dilemmas – is consciousness lost, or simply no longer apparent? This question is at the heart of, *Coma and Disorders of Consciousness* edited by Caroline Schnakers and Steven Laureys of the Coma Science Group based at the University of Liège. The Coma Science Group is one of the most prolific and accomplished research teams currently engaged in the study of patients with disorders of consciousness (DoC). Laureys and Schnakers, specifically, are responsible for many seminal papers in this rapidly advancing field. Together, they have assembled an outstanding list of authors, most associated with the Coma Science Group, and have compiled a comprehensive volume that aptly depicts the state of the science in assessment and treatment of patients with DoC. The first half of the book is devoted to technological advances in diagnostic and prognostic assessment, appropriately reflecting the most important developments over the last 5 years. Novel applications of functional neuroimaging (i.e., fMRI) and electrophysiologic (i.e., EEG, ERP) methods of detecting conscious awareness in behaviourally non-responsive patients are addressed, as are imaging techniques that index brain metabolites (i.e., spectroscopy), white matter tracts (i.e., diffusion tensor imaging) and patterns of neural activation (i.e., transcranial magnetic stimulation), which may be of prognostic significance. The second half of the book focuses largely on treatment interventions ranging from sensory stimulation to neuromodulation strategies (i.e., pharmacotherapy, deep brain stimulation, brain computer interface). Two important but understudied areas, sleep and oral feeding, are also covered. The book concludes with a discussion of the ethical conundrums associated with clinical management of patients with DoC and a forward look at this pivotal area of discovery, located at the crossroads of philosophy and science. This book continues the search for the "seat of consciousness" begun more than two millennia ago – a quest that, by virtue of the human condition, we are compelled to undertake. For this reason, no reader will turn away from this book disappointed.

Harvard Medical School, Boston, MA, USA Joseph T. Giacino

Foreword II

The definition of "*the persistent vegetative state*" by Jennett and Plum in 1972 constituted an important step in the understanding and the monitoring of patients presenting a disorder of consciousness after a period of coma. However, for years, the scientific work on this topic remained insignificant. The merit of the Coma Science Group is to have been interested in these patients with a new perspective, at a clinical but also scientific and ethical level. These researchers are using tools of modern neuroscience, particularly, functional neuroimaging and electrophysiology, in order to better understand the brain functioning of patients recovering from coma. They showed, for instance, that patients diagnosed as being in a "*vegetative*" state could present conscious activity unsuspected at a clinical level. Their approach did not remain only theoretical, as they were also interested in clinical assessment and, particularly, in the risk of diagnostic errors, in the care and in the complex ethical problems associated with these vulnerable patients. This team, in parallel with British researchers, significantly contributed to the progress of knowledge in this field. This book coordinated by Steven Laureys and Caroline Schnakers presents a complete review of the main clinical and scientific advances on the disorders of consciousness, including a synthesis of their own work. It also tackles questions about the future, such as pharmacological treatment or deep brain stimulation. Ethical questions are also discussed. I am sure that this book, coordinated by two of the best experts in the field, will meet the success it deserves and will quickly become a classic for all clinicians and researchers working with these patients.

Université de Versailles-Saint Quentin, Garches, France

Philippe Azouvi

Preface

Consciousness is a word worn smooth by a million tongues. Depending upon the figure of speech chosen it is a state of being, a substance, a process, a place, an epiphenomenon, an emergent aspect of matter, or the only true reality.

George Armitage Miller

Fifty years ago, the field of disorders of consciousness was a very limited research domain. Severely brain-injured patients, who are most likely to present impaired consciousness during recovery, often died. In the 1950s, the introduction of artificial breathing changed everything. The life of these patients could be extended even in cases of severe lesions to brain areas supporting the control of vital functions. The clinician started to face patients who were alive but not reactive to their surroundings. In this context, a new field was called to emerge. In the 1960s, Plum and Posner defined for the first time a clinical entity called the coma. Slightly later, Jennett and Teasdale developed the well-known Glasgow Coma Scale for assessing the progress of comatose patients in intensive care units. The 1980s were characterized by the development of a new kind of treatment, the sensory stimulation programs. In the late 1990s, the emergence of neuroimaging techniques opened new opportunities to study brain reactivity in patients with disorders of consciousness.

However, in spite of the medical advances and the increasing number of severely brain-injured patients, the assessment and treatment of patients recovering from coma represents a very difficult and delicate task even today. The detection of signs of consciousness is complicated by the frequent motor and cognitive limitations of these patients. Treatment options are nearly absent, leaving the clinician often with a situation of palliative rather than restorative care. Even in an experimental setting, the study of patients in a coma or related disorders of consciousness is a real challenge. These patients are easily exhausted, limiting the assessment window, and spontaneous motor reactions have to be controlled for. The development of a research environment adapted to the scientific investigation of these patients is time consuming and requests important clinical and scientific expertise. For over 10 years now, the Coma Science Group (http://www.coma.ulg.ac.be) has been working on the scientific exploration of disorders of consciousness, with both scientific and clinical research agendas. This research team, bridging various medical (neurology, neurosurgery, intensive care, anesthesia, physical medicine, otorhinolaryngology) and paramedical disciplines (psychology, speech therapy, physical therapy) as well as engineering and biological disciplines, has been a major player in the development of new assessment, communication, and treatment techniques for disorders of consciousness, and this at both the behavioral and the neuroimaging level. We decided to write this book in order to offer clinicians as well as researchers an overview of the most recent advancements in this domain.

By focusing on both clinicians and researchers as potential readers of this book, we decided to include well-established findings about diagnostic/prognostic criteria, ethical issues, assessment techniques (i.e., behavioral scales, electrophysiological explorations, and structural/functional neuroimaging), and treatment procedures, but also techniques under development (i.e., the use of classifiers, brain-computer interfaces, transcranial magnetic stimulation, or deep brain stimulation) which, we hope, will stimulate ideas for future research.

In conclusion, we hope to have reached our aim by offering a comprehensive and reader-friendly book to readers both familiar or not with the difficult but intriguing field of disorders of consciousness.

We hope you enjoy reading this book.

University of Liège, Liège, Belgium

Caroline Schnakers
Steven Laureys

Acknowledgment

Our work is supported by the National Funds for Scientific Research (FRS), James S. McDonnell Foundation, Mind Science Foundation Texas, US National Institutes of Health, European Commission (Mindbridge, DISCOS, DECODER & COST), French Speaking Community Concerted Research Action, Belgian Federal Public Service of Health, Fonds Leon Fredericq, Public Utility Foundation "Université Européenne du Travail," "Fondazione Europea di Ricerca Biomedica," and the University and University Hospital of Liège.

Contents

Contributors

Philippe Azouvi, M.D., Ph.D. Department of Neurological Rehabilitation, AP-HP, Hôpital Raymond-Poincaré; Université de Versailles-Saint Quentin, Garches, France

Melanie Boly, M.D., Ph.D. Coma Science Group, Cyclotron Research Center, University of Liège, Liège, Belgium

Ingrid Breuskin, M.D., Ph.D. Oto-Rhino-Laryngology Head and Neck Surgery Department, University Hospital of Liège, Liège, Belgium

Marie-Aurélie Bruno, Ph.D. Coma Science Group, Cyclotron Research Center, University of Liège, Liège, Belgium

Vanessa Charland-Verville, M.Sc. Coma Science Group, Cyclotron Research Center, University of Liège, Liège, Belgium

Camille Chatelle, M.Sc. Coma Science Group, Cyclotron Research Center, University of Liège, Liège, Belgium

Victor Cologan, M.Sc. Coma Science Group, Cyclotron Research Center, University of Liège, Liège, Belgium

Athena Demertzi, M.Sc. Coma Science Group, Cyclotron Research Center, University of Liège, Liège, Belgium

Haibo Di, Ph.D. Physiology Department, International Vegetative State and Consciousness Science Institute, Hangzhou Normal University, Hangzhou, China

Joseph T. Giacino, Ph.D. Department of Physical Medicine and Rehabilitation Medicine, Spaulding Rehabilitation Hospital/Harvard Medical School, Boston, MA, USA

Olivia Gosseries, M.Sc. Coma Science Group, Cyclotron Research Center, University of Liège, Liège, Belgium

Murielle Kirsch, M.D. Coma Science Group, Cyclotron Research Center, University of Liège, Liège, Belgium

Department of Anesthesiology, University Hospital of Liège, Liège, Belgium

Steven Laureys, M.D., Ph.D. Coma Science Group, Cyclotron Research Center, University of Liège, Liège, Belgium

Department of Neurology, University Hospital of Liège, Liège, Belgium

Didier Ledoux, M.D. Coma Science Group, Cyclotron Research Center, University of Liège, Liège, Belgium

Department of Intensive Care, University Hospital of Liège, Liège, Belgium

Rémy Lehembre, M.Sc. Coma Science Group, Cyclotron Research Center, University of Liège, Liège, Belgium

Zulay Lugo, M.Sc. Coma Science Group, Cyclotron Research Center, University of Liège, Liège, Belgium

Department of Psychology, Biological Psychology, Clinical Psychology and Psychotherapy, University of Würzburg, Würzburg, Germany

Dorothee Lulé, Ph.D. Section of Neurophysiology, Department of Neurology, University of Ulm, Ulm, Germany

Steve Majerus, Ph.D. Coma Science Group, Cyclotron Research Center, University of Liège, Liège, Belgium

Marcello Massimini, Ph.D. Physiology Department, University of Milan, Milan, Italy

Audrey Maudoux, M.D. Oto-Rhino-Laryngology Head and Neck Surgery Department, University Hospital of Liège, Liège, Belgium

Coma Science Group, Cyclotron Research Center, University of Liège, Liège, Belgium

Quentin Noirhomme, Ph.D. Coma Science Group, Cyclotron Research Center, University of Liège, Liège, Belgium

Christophe L.M. Phillips, Ph.D. Cyclotron Research Center, University of Liège, Liège, Belgium

Mario Rosanova, Ph.D. Physiology Department, University of Milan, Milan, Italy

Manuel Schabus, Ph.D. Department of Psychology, Laboratory for Sleep and Consciousness Research, University of Salzburg, Salzburg, Austria

Caroline Schnakers, Ph.D. Coma Science Group, Cyclotron Research Center, University of Liège, Liège, Belgium

Jessica Schrouff, M.Sc. Cyclotron Research Center, University of Liège, Liège, Belgium

Andrea Soddu, Ph.D. Coma Science Group, Cyclotron Research Center, University of Liège, Liège, Belgium

Bettina Sorger, Ph.D. Coma Science Group, Cyclotron Research Center, University of Liège, Liège, Belgium

Department of Cognitive Neuroscience, Faculty of Psychology and Neuroscience, Maastricht University and Maastricht Brain Imaging Centre (M-BIC), Maastricht, The Netherlands

Aurore Thibaut, M.Sc. Coma Science Group, Cyclotron Research Center, University of Liège, Liège, Belgium

Marie Thonnard, M.Sc. Coma Science Group, Cyclotron Research Center, University of Liège, Liège, Belgium

Jean-Flory Luaba Tshibanda, M.D. Coma Science Group, Cyclotron Research Center, University of Liège, Liège, Belgium

Department of Radiology, University Hospital of Liège, Liège, Belgium

Audrey Vanhaudenhuyse, Ph.D. Coma Science Group, Cyclotron Research Center, University of Liège, Liège, Belgium

Chapter 1
Behavioral Assessment and Diagnosis of Disorders of Consciousness

Caroline Schnakers and Steve Majerus

Introduction

During these last years, there has been increasing fascination for the field of disorders of consciousness. Due to progress in intensive care, more and more severely brain-injured patients survive their initial brain insult, but many of these will go through various states of impaired consciousness. The proportion of these patients is estimated at 46 per million in the United States, 14 per million in Great Britain [1], and 36 per million in Belgium [2]. Many patients will remain in a vegetative state for a more or less extended period of time before regaining some level of consciousness (minimally conscious state). Some of these cases have been widely broadcasted, such as the case of Terri Shiavo (1963–2005) who stayed in a vegetative state for 15 years after a cardiac arrest or the case of Terry Wallis who emerged from a minimally conscious state 19 years (1984–2003) after a severe traumatic brain injury [3]. At the same time, prolonged hospitalization is expensive. In the United States, the costs are estimated between 600,000 and 1,875,000 dollars per year per patient with severe traumatic injury [4]. Questions regarding end-of-life decisions are critical here, particularly in chronic vegetative patients. In a recent European survey ($n = 2{,}475$), the majority of medical and paramedical professionals

C. Schnakers, Ph.D. (✉)
Coma Science Group, Cyclotron Research Center, University of Liège,
Allée du 6 Août, Sart Tilman B30, 4000 Liège, Belgium
e-mail: c.schnakers@ulg.ac.be

S. Majerus, Ph.D.
Coma Science Group, Cyclotron Research Center, University of Liège,
Allée du 6 Août, Sart Tilman B30, 4000 Liège, Belgium

Department of Psychology, Cognition and Behavior, University of Liège,
Boulevard du Rectorat 3 B33, 4000 Liège, Belgium
e-mail: smajerus@ulg.ac.be

C. Schnakers, S. Laureys (eds.), *Coma and Disorders of Consciousness*,
DOI 10.1007/978-1-4471-2440-5_1, © Springer-Verlag London 2012

(66%) agreed to withdraw life support for chronic vegetative patients while only 28% agreed for patients in a chronic minimally conscious state. Many clinicians reported that they would not want to be life-supported if they happened themselves to be in a chronic vegetative state (82%) or if they were in a chronic minimally conscious state (67%) [5]. As we can see, the social, economic, and ethical consequences associated with disorders of consciousness, and particularly the vegetative state, are gigantic.

The term "*vegetative*" indicates preserved physiological functions (cardiac, respiratory, sleep/wake cycles) without clear signs of consciousness of either the self or the environment. In a sense, the body works without the mind. One of the few ways we have to differentiate these patients from conscious patients is to observe their spontaneous behaviors and their reactions to stimuli occurring in their environment. This behavioral assessment requests thorough expertise on behalf of the clinician. It also depends on the physical and mental capacities (particularly, the vigilance level) of the patient at the time of assessment. Missing signs of consciousness is not a rare fact, and diagnostic errors are frequent (i.e., around 40%) [6–8]. The diagnosis is, however, crucial. It influences the way the patient's care will be oriented and the way end-of-life decisions will be considered with the patient's family. Developing valid and sensitive behavioral scales to detect the presence of signs of consciousness, even subtle, therefore, represents a real challenge.

Disorders of Consciousness: Definition

We present here the different states of altered consciousness (i.e., brain death, coma, vegetative state and minimally conscious state) that can occur in severely brain-injured patients (Table 1.1).

Brain Death

In brain death, the organism does not function anymore without medical assistance [9, 10]. Critical functions such as respiration, blood circulation, neuroendocrine, and homeostatic regulation are absent. The patient is apneic and unreactive to environmental stimulation. The term "*brain death*" requires the demonstration of irreversible cessation of all clinical functions of the brain, but also, of the brainstem [11]. Brain death is classically caused by a brain lesion (e.g., massive traumatic injury, intracranial hemorrhage, or anoxia) that results in increased intracranial pressure (i.e., higher than the mean arterial blood pressure). The diagnosis can be made within 6–24 h postinjury [12].

Table 1.1 Diagnostic criteria for brain death, coma, vegetative, and minimally conscious states and locked-in syndrome

Consciousness level	Diagnostic criteria
Brain death	No arousal/eye-opening
	No behavioral signs of awareness
	Apnea
	Loss of brain functions (brainstem reflexes)
Coma	No arousal/eye-opening
	No behavioral signs of awareness
	Impaired spontaneous breathing
	Impaired brainstem reflexes
	No vocalizations
	>1 h
Vegetative state	Arousal/spontaneous or stimulus-induced eye opening
	No behavioral signs of awareness
	Preserved spontaneous breathing
	Preserved brainstem reflexes
	No purposeful behaviors
	No language production or comprehension
	Preservation (partial or complete) of hypothalamic and brain stem autonomic functions
	Preservation of sleep-wake cycle
	>1 month: persistent vegetative
	Compatible:
	Grimaces to pain
	Localization to sounds
	Atypical but compatible:
	Visual fixation
	Response to threat
	Inappropriate single words
Minimally conscious state	Arousal/spontaneous eye-opening
	Fluctuating but reproducible behavioral signs of awareness
	Response to verbal order
	Environmentally-contingent smiling or crying
	Object localization and manipulation
	Sustained visual fixation and pursuit
	Verbalizations
	Intentional but unreliable communication
	Emergence from MCS:
	Functional communication
	Functional object use
Locked-in syndrome	Arousal/spontaneous eye-opening
	Preserved cognitive functions
	Communication via eye gaze
	Anarthria
	Tetraplegia

Coma

Brain injured patients can stay in coma for several weeks, showing no arousal or awareness; the eyes are constantly closed and no voluntary behavioral responses are observed [13]. In most cases, patients emerge from their comatose state within 2–4 weeks postinjury. The prognosis for recovery is influenced by different factors such as etiology, the patient's general medical condition, and age. Outcome is known to be unfavorable if, during 3 consecutive days, there are no pupillary or corneal reflexes, stereotyped or absent motor responses to noxious stimulation, and isoelectrical or burst suppression EEG patterns [14]. Prognosis for recovery in traumatic coma survivors is better than in anoxic cases. Recovery from coma may lead to a vegetative state, a minimally conscious state or, more rarely, to a locked-in syndrome.

Vegetative State

The term "*vegetative state*" (VS) was defined to describe "*an organic body capable of growth and development but devoid of sensation and thought*" [1]. This state implies the preservation of autonomic functions (e.g., cardiovascular regulation, thermoregulation) and sleep–wake cycles in the absence of awareness. Behaviorally, patients in VS open their eyes spontaneously or in response to stimulation, but they only show reflex behaviors, unrelated to the environment [15]. It is very important to stress the difference between persistent and permanent VS, which are – both being referred to as PVS – causing unnecessary confusion. When the term "*persistent vegetative state*" was first described, it was emphasized that persistent did not mean permanent; it is now recommended to omit "*persistent*" and to mention the time during which a patient has been in a VS. In the absence of recovery after a specified period (i.e., 3 months for traumatic etiology and 12 months for nontraumatic etiologies) the state can be declared to be permanent and, only then, the ethical and legal issues concerning treatment withdrawal can be discussed [16]. Given the negative connotation of the term "*vegetative state*", it has been recently proposed to use the term "*unresponsive wakefulness syndrome*" rather than "*vegetative state*" [17].

Minimally Conscious State

Patients in a minimally conscious state (MCS) are awake and show fluctuating but reproducible signs of awareness. These patients can manifest emotional and oriented behavioral responses such as response to verbal order, object manipulation, oriented responses to noxious stimulation, visual pursuit, or fixation. However, these behaviors can fluctuate in time, which makes the detection of awareness a difficult endeavor. Recovery from MCS is defined by the emergence of functional communication and/or functional object use. Even if prognosis is better as compared to VS, some patients can remain in an MCS without fully recovering consciousness for a prolonged period of time [18].

Locked-in Syndrome

The Locked-in Syndrome (LIS) is *not* a disorder of consciousness, although it may present as one. Misdiagnosis is very frequent here [19]. LIS patients cannot move or talk due to quadriplegia; only vertical eye movements and eye blinking may be used to communicate with their environment. Typically, the diagnosis of LIS is not established until 2.5 months post-onset. There are reports suggesting that family members tend to detect signs of consciousness prior to medical staff [20]. This syndrome is often due to a selective supranuclear motor de-efferentation, producing a paralysis of all four limbs and the last cranial nerves without interfering with consciousness or cognition. According to Bauer et al. [21], different categories of LIS can be distinguished based on the extent of motor impairment: (1) *Classical* LIS consists of a total immobility but preserved vertical eye movements and blinking; (2) *Incomplete* LIS is characterized by remnant nonocular voluntary motions (e.g., head or fingers movements); (3) *Total* LIS patients are completely immobile, unable to control any eye movement, and nearly impossible to diagnose before the development of neuroimaging [21]. Patients with LIS may live for 12 or more years while remaining in this state of complete immobility [22]. It is important to note that LIS patients rate their quality of life to be similar to the quality of life in the healthy population [23]. In the absence of other structural or functional brain abnormalities, patients with LIS are fully able to make their own decisions [24].

Behavioral Scales

Behavioral observation constitutes the major tool for detecting signs of consciousness in severely brain injured patients. The detection of voluntary behaviors is nevertheless difficult and signs of consciousness can easily be missed due to sensory and motor disabilities, tracheostomy, fluctuating arousal levels, or ambiguous and rapidly exhausted responses. Numerous behavioral rating scales have been developed and validated to assess levels of consciousness and to help establishing accurate diagnoses. We have to distinguish here "*arousal*" from "*consciousness*." Indeed, a patient can be aroused but show no signs of consciousness, as in VS. Preservation of arousal is, therefore, a necessary but insufficient condition for consciousness (Fig. 1.1) [25]. In this section, we briefly review commonly used behavioral instruments for the assessment of consciousness.

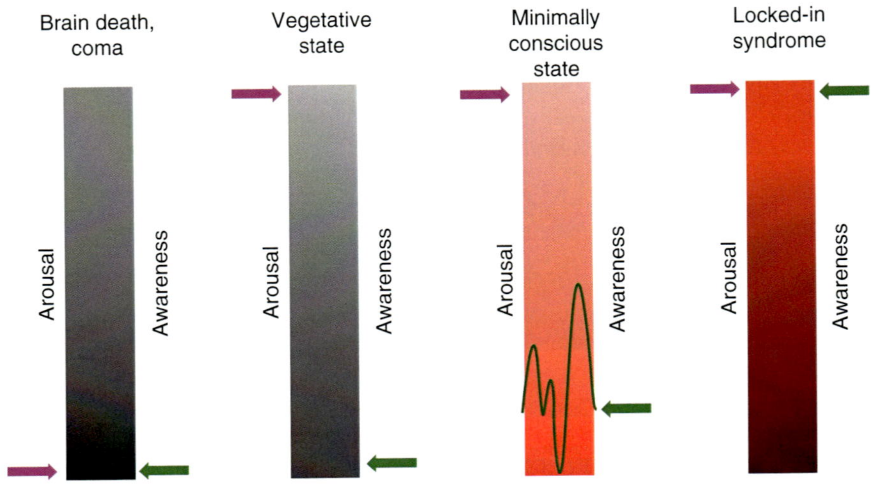

Fig. 1.1 Behavioral observation assesses two dimensions of consciousness: arousal and awareness. In brain death and coma, both dimensions are absent. In the vegetative state, arousal level is relatively preserved in the absence of signs of awareness. In the minimally conscious state, both dimensions are present although behavioral signs often fluctuate. In the locked-in syndrome, both dimensions are fully preserved despite complete loss of speech and motor functions

The Glasgow Coma Scale (GCS)

The GCS [26, 27] remains the most widely used tool in traumatic and acute-care settings. The GCS was the first validated rating scale developed to monitor levels of consciousness in the intensive care unit. This scale is relatively brief and can be easily incorporated into routine clinical care. It includes three subscales that address arousal level, motor function, and verbal abilities. Subscale scores are added and yield a total score ranging from 3 to 15. The GCS has been extensively investigated for its prognostic value [28]. Despite its widespread use, the GCS has been criticized for variable inter-rater agreement and problems in deriving scores in patients with ocular trauma, tracheostomy, or ventilatory support [29–34].

The Full Outline of UnResponsiveness Scale (FOUR)

The FOUR was recently developed to replace the GCS to assess severely brain-injured patients in intensive care [35–37]. The scale includes four subscales assessing motor and ocular responses, brainstem reflexes, and breathing. The total score ranges from 0 to 16. Unlike the GCS, the FOUR does not assess verbal functions to accommodate the high number of intubated patients in intensive care.

A score of 0 on the FOUR assumes the absence of brainstem reflexes and breathing and, therefore, helps to diagnose brain death. The scale also monitors recovery of autonomic functions and tracks emergence from VS. The FOUR is specifically designed to detect patients in a locked-in syndrome as it uses oculomotor commands that detect vertical eye movements and eye blinks, both being preserved in LIS.

The Wessex Head Injury Matrix (WHIM)

The WHIM [38, 39] was developed to capture changes in patients in VS until emergence from posttraumatic amnesia. This tool is particularly sensitive to detecting changes in patients in MCS not captured by traditional scales such as the GCS. Shiel et al. longitudinally followed 97 severely brain injured patients recovering from coma to create the WHIM. The 62-items were ordered according to the mean sequence of recovery observed in these patients; they assess arousal level and concentration, visual consciousness (i.e., visual pursuit), communication, cognition (i.e., memory and spatiotemporal orientation), and social behaviors. The WHIM score represents the rank of the most complex behavior observed [40].

The JFK Coma Recovery Scale (CRS-R)

The CRS-R was originally developed by investigators from the JFK Johnson Rehabilitation Institute in 1991. The scale was revised and published in 2004 as the JFK Coma Recovery Scale-Revised (CRS-R) [41–46]. The purpose of the CRS-R is to assist with differential diagnosis, prognostic assessment, and treatment planning in patients with disorders of consciousness. The scale consists of 23 items that comprise six subscales addressing auditory, visual, motor, oromotor, communication, and arousal functions. CRS-R subscales are comprised of hierarchically-arranged items associated with brain stem, subcortical, and cortical processes. The lowest item on each subscale represents reflexive activity while the highest items represent cognitively mediated behaviors. Scoring is standardized and based on the presence or absence of operationally defined behavioral responses to specific sensory stimuli. Psychometric studies indicate that the CRS-R meets minimal standards for measurement and evaluation tools designed for use in interdisciplinary medical rehabilitation. The CRS-R can be administered reliably by trained examiners and produces reasonably stable scores over repeated assessments. Validity analyses have shown that the CRS-R is capable of discriminating patients in MCS from those in VS, which is of critical importance in establishing prognosis and formulating treatment interventions [42, 44].

Pain Assessment: The Nociception Coma Scale

Patients recovering from coma are unable to communicate their feelings and their perception of pain. It is, hence, important to develop sensitive instruments to assess pain perception in these patients. Even if pain scales were developed to assess pain in different types of noncommunicative populations (such as demented elderly and newborns), none of these are adapted to detect pain in severely brain-injured patients. In this context, the Nociception Coma Scale (NCS) was recently developed [47, 48]. This scale includes the observation of motor, verbal, and visual responses as well as facial expression following pain. The total score varies from 0 to 12. A validation study of the NCS was performed by observing the responses of 48 VS and MCS patients following a nociceptive stimulation (pressure applied to the bed of the fingernail). Results showed a good inter-rater agreement and concurrent validity between NCS and other pain scales validated for demented elderly patients and newborns. However, in contrast to these scales, the total score of the NCS significantly differed according to the level of consciousness, with higher scores in MCS versus VS patients, suggesting that the scale is particularly adapted to assess pain in patients recovering from coma. These results show that the NCS is a sensitive scale, which specifically assesses pain in noncommunicative severely brain-injured patients.

Conclusion

Accurately diagnosing patients with a disorder of consciousness represents a real challenge. A recent study showed that about 40% of patients clinically diagnosed as being in a vegetative state present, in fact, signs of consciousness [8]. The recovery of consciousness is usually gradual, sometimes marked by clear signs of consciousness, but more often these signs are subtle. The assessment of residual cognitive functioning is complicated by vigilance fluctuations, motor deficits, and other confounding factors. The knowledge of diagnostic criteria and the use of valid and sensitive standardized scales are, therefore, essential to establish a precise diagnosis.

References

1. Jennett B. 30 years of the vegetative state: clinical, ethical and legal problems. In: Laureys S, editor. The boundaries of consciousness: neurobiology and neuropathology, vol. 150. Amsterdam: Elsevier; 2005. p. 541–8.
2. Demotte R. Politique de la santé à mener à l'égard des patients en état végétatif persistant ou en état pauci-relationnel. Moniteur Belge. 2004;69334–40.
3. Wijdicks EF. Minimally conscious state vs. persistent vegetative state: the case of Terry (Wallis) vs. the case of Terri (Schiavo). Mayo Clin Proc. 2006;81(9):1155–8.

4. Consensus conference. Rehabilitation of persons with traumatic brain injury. NIH consensus development panel on rehabilitation of persons with traumatic brain injury. JAMA. 1999;282(10):974–83.
5. Demertzi A, Ledoux D, Bruno MA, et al. Attitudes towards end-of-life issues in disorders of consciousness: a European survey. J Neurol. 2011;258:1058–65.
6. Childs NL, Mercer WN, Childs HW. Accuracy of diagnosis of persistent vegetative state. Neurology. 1993;43(8):1465–7.
7. Andrews K, Murphy L, Munday R, Littlewood C. Misdiagnosis of the vegetative state: retrospective study in a rehabilitation unit. BMJ. 1996;313(7048):13–6.
8. Schnakers C, Vanhaudenhuyse A, Giacino J, et al. Diagnostic accuracy of the vegetative and minimally conscious state: clinical consensus versus standardized neurobehavioral assessment. BMC Neurol. 2009;9:35.
9. Bernat JL. A defense of the whole-brain concept of death. Hastings Cent Rep. 1998;28(2): 14–23.
10. Haupt WF, Rudolf J. European brain death codes: a comparison of national guidelines. J Neurol. 1999;246(6):432–7.
11. Pallis C, Harley DH. ABC of brainstem death. 2nd ed. London: BMJ Publishing Group; 1996.
12. Medical Consultants on the Diagnosis of Death. Guidelines for the determination of death. Report of the medical consultants on the diagnosis of death to the President's Commission for the Study of Ethical Problems in Medicine and Biomedical and Behavioral Research. JAMA. 1981;246(19):2184–6.
13. Plum F, Posner JB. The diagnosis of stupor and coma. 1st ed. Philadelphia: Davis, F.A; 1966.
14. Attia J, Cook DJ. Prognosis in anoxic and traumatic coma. Crit Care Clin. 1998;14(3):497–511.
15. The Multi-Society Task Force on PVS. Medical aspects of the persistent vegetative state (1). N Engl J Med. 1994;330(21):1499–508.
16. Monti M, Laureys S, Owen A. The vegetative state. BMJ. 2010;341:3765.
17. Laureys S, Celesia G, Cohadon F, et al. Unresponsive wakefulness syndrome: a new name for the vegetative state or apallic syndrome. BMC Med. 2010;8(1):68.
18. Giacino J, Ashwal S, Childs N, et al. The minimally conscious state: definition and diagnostic criteria. Neurology. 2002;58(3):349–53.
19. American Congress of Rehabilitation Medicine. Recommendations for use of uniform nomenclature pertinent to patients with severe alterations of consciousness. Arch Phys Med Rehabil. 1995;76:205–9.
20. Laureys S, Pellas F, Van Eeckhout P, et al. The locked-in syndrome: what is it like to be conscious but paralyzed and voiceless? Prog Brain Res. 2005;150:495–511.
21. Bauer G, Gerstenbrand F, Rumpl E. Varieties of the locked-in syndrome. J Neurol. 1979;221(2):77–91.
22. Katz RT, Haig AJ, Clark BB, DiPaola RJ. Long-term survival, prognosis, and life-care planning for 29 patients with chronic locked-in syndrome. Arch Phys Med Rehabil. 1992;73(5):403–8.
23. Lule D, Zickler C, Hacker S, et al. Life can be worth living in locked-in syndrome. Prog Brain Res. 2009;177:339–51.
24. Bruno M, Bernheim JL, Schnakers C, Laureys S. Locked-in: don't judge a book by its cover. J Neurol Neurosurg Psychiatry. 2008;79(1):2.
25. Majerus S, Gill-Thwaites H, Andrews K, Laureys S. Behavioral evaluation of consciousness in severe brain damage. In: Laureys S, editor. The boundaries of consciousness: neurobiology and neuropathology. Amsterdam: Elsevier; 2005. p. 397–413.
26. Teasdale G, Jennett B. Assessment of coma and impaired consciousness. A practical scale. Lancet. 1974;2(7872):81–4.
27. Teasdale G. Acute impairment of brain function-1. Assessing 'conscious level'. Nurs Times. 1975;71(24):914–7.

28. McNett M. A review of the predictive ability of Glasgow Coma Scale scores in head-injured patients. J Neurosci Nurs. 2007;39(2):68–75.
29. Jagger J, Jane JA, Rimel R. The Glasgow Coma Scale: to sum or not to sum? Lancet. 1983;2(8341):97.
30. Koziol JA, Hacke W. Multivariate data reduction by principal components, with application to neurological scoring instruments. J Neurol. 1990;237(8):461–4.
31. Rowley G, Fielding K. Reliability and accuracy of the Glasgow Coma Scale with experienced and inexperienced users. Lancet. 1991;337(8740):535–8.
32. Moskopp D, Stähle C, Wassermann HD. Problems of the Glasgow Coma Scale with early intubated patients. Neurosurg Rev. 1995;18:253–7.
33. Wijdicks EF, Kokmen E, O'Brien PC. Measurement of impaired consciousness in the neurological intensive care unit: a new test. J Neurol Neurosurg Psychiatry. 1998;64:117–9.
34. Bhatty GB, Kapoor N. The Glasgow Coma Scale: a mathematical critique. Acta Neurochir. 1993;120(3–4):132–5.
35. Wijdicks EF. Clinical scales for comatose patients: the Glasgow Coma Scale in historical context and the new FOUR score. Rev Neurol Dis. 2006;3(3):109–17.
36. Wijdicks EF, Bamlet WR, Maramattom BV, et al. Validation of a new coma scale: the FOUR score. Ann Neurol. 2005;58(4):585–93.
37. Bruno MA, Ledoux D, Lambermont B, et al. Comparison of the full outline of UnResponsiveness and Glasgow liege scale/Glasgow Coma Scale in an intensive care unit population. Neurocrit Care. 2011;15(3):447–53.
38. Shiel A, Horn SA, Wilson BA, et al. The wessex head injury matrix (WHIM) main scale: a preliminary report on a scale to assess and monitor patient recovery after severe head injury. Clin Rehabil. 2000;14(4):408–16.
39. Majerus S, Van der Linden M. Wessex head injury matrix and Glasgow/Glasgow-liège Coma Scale: a validation and comparison study. Neuropsychol Rehabil. 2000;10(2):167–84.
40. Wilson FC, Elder V, McCrudden E, Caldwell S. Analysis of wessex head injury matrix (WHIM) scores in consecutive vegetative and minimally conscious state patients. Neuropsychol Rehabil. 2009;19(5):754–60.
41. Giacino J, Kalmar K, Whyte J. The JFK coma recovery scale-revised: measurement characteristics and diagnostic utility. Arch Phys Med Rehabil. 2004;85(12):2020–9.
42. Schnakers C, Majerus S, Giacino J, et al. A French validation study of the coma recovery scale-revised (CRS-R). Brain Inj. 2008;22(10):786–92.
43. Lovstad M, Froslie KF, Giacino JT, et al. Reliability and diagnostic characteristics of the JFK coma recovery scale-revised: exploring the influence of rater's level of experience. J Head Trauma Rehabil. 2010;25(5):349–56.
44. Schnakers C, Giacino J, Kalmar K, et al. Does the FOUR score correctly diagnose the vegetative and minimally conscious states? Ann Neurol. 2006;60(6):744–5.
45. Seel RT, Sherer M, Whyte J, et al. Assessment scales for disorders of consciousness: evidence-based recommendations for clinical practice and research. Arch Phys Med Rehabil. 2010;91(12):1795–813.
46. Giacino J, Kezmarsky MA, DeLuca J, Cicerone KD. Monitoring rate of recovery to predict outcome in minimally responsive patients. Arch Phys Med Rehabil. 1991;72(11):897–901.
47. Schnakers C, Chatelle C, Vanhaudenhuyse A, et al. The nociception coma scale: a new tool to assess nociception in disorders of consciousness. Pain. 2010;148(2):215–9.
48. Schnakers C, Chatelle C, Majerus S, et al. Assessment and detection of pain in non-communicative severely brain-injured patients. Expert Rev Neurother. 2010;10(11):1725–31.

Chapter 2
Prognosis of Patients with Altered State of Consciousness

Marie-Aurélie Bruno, Didier Ledoux, Audrey Vanhaudenhuyse, Olivia Gosseries, Aurore Thibaut, and Steven Laureys

Introduction

Medical technologies and treatment developments led to an increase in patients surviving severe brain damage. A patient's prognosis is important not only for the patient, but also for his family, as well as for the caregivers. The family has to deal with the patient's cognitive and motor deficits caused by the accident, the lack of communication, and the emotions associated with the events. Healthcare profes-

M.-A. Bruno, Ph.D. (✉) • A. Vanhaudenhuyse, Ph.D. •
A. Thibaut, M.Sc. • S. Laureys, M.D., Ph.D.
Coma Science Group, Cyclotron Research Center, University of Liège,
Allée du 6 Août, Sart Tilman B30, 4000 Liège, Belgium

Department of Neurology, University Hospital of Liège,
Liège, Belgium
e-mail: ma.bruno@ulg.ac.be; avanhaudenhuyse@ulg.ac.be; athibaut@ulg.ac.be; steven.laureys@ulg.ac.be

D. Ledoux, M.D.
Coma Science Group, Cyclotron Research Center, University of Liège,
Allée du 6 Août, Sart Tilman B30, 4000 Liège, Belgium

Department of Intensive Care, University Hospital of Liège,
Liège, Belgium

Department of Neurology, University Hospital of Liège,
Liège, Belgium
e-mail: dledoux@chu.ulg.ac.be

O. Gosseries, M.Sc.
Coma Science Group, Cyclotron Research Center, University of Liège,
Allée du 6 Août, Sart Tilman B30, 4000 Liège, Belgium

Department of Neurology, University Hospital of Liège,
Liège, Belgium

National Fund for Scientific Research, Liège, Belgium
e-mail: ogosseries@ulg.ac.be

C. Schnakers, S. Laureys (eds.), *Coma and Disorders of Consciousness*,
DOI 10.1007/978-1-4471-2440-5_2, © Springer-Verlag London 2012

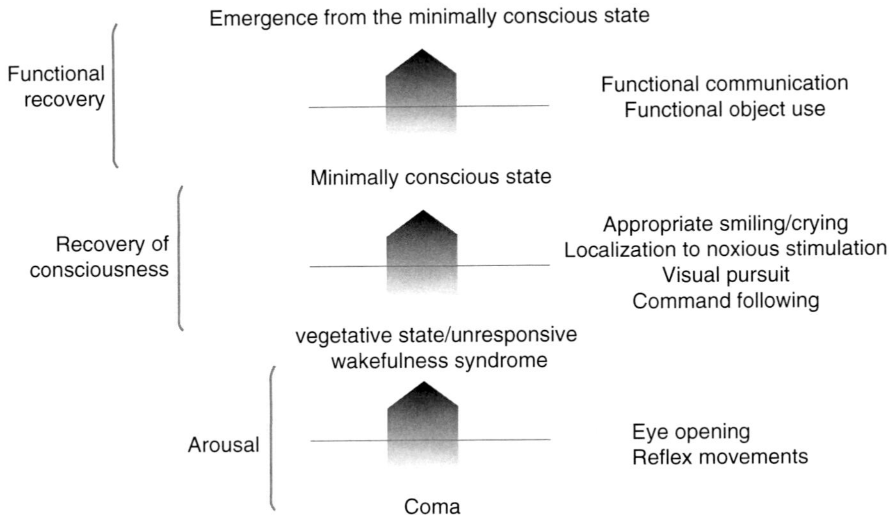

Fig. 2.1 Behaviorally progressive transitions from coma, to vegetative state/unresponsive wakefulness syndrome, to minimally conscious state, to emergence from the minimally conscious state

sionals are involved in the daily care, in assessing the effectiveness of various medical treatments, and in any end-of-life decisions. A patient's recovery can be considered according to three dimensions: survival/mortality, recovery of consciousness (minimally conscious state – MCS), and functional recovery (the emergence from MCS). Several factors are associated with an increased mortality in patients with altered state of consciousness: (1) a Glasgow motor scale ≤2 [1], (2) the absence of pupillary and/or corneal reflex, (3) a status epilepticus, (4) an isoelectric EEG ("flat EEG"), (5) the absence of Somatosensory Evoked Potentials (N20), and (6) an increased serum concentration of neuron-specific enolase (NSE) [2–4].

Medical complications such as hypotension, hyperthermia, hyperglycemia, infections, or prolonged mechanical ventilation also decrease the chances of survival [4–6]. Most common causes of death in the intensive care and rehabilitation units are urinary and pulmonary infections, heart failure and cachexia, sudden death, and organ failure [7, 8]. After the acute phase and once medical complications are stabilized, the potential degree of recovery should be evaluated. Patients may show signs of consciousness recovery or functional recovery. Recovery of consciousness can be translated by the presence of clear-cut signs of self- or environmental awareness (fluctuating voluntary responses to a verbal and/or a written request, visual tracking, context-specific emotional responses, etc. – MCS) [9]. Functional recovery is characterized by the recuperation of a functional communication and/or a functional use of objects and/or an ability to learn and perform new tasks as well as to participate in personal, professional, or recreational activities (emergence from MCS) [10]. Recovery of consciousness can occur without functional recovery. Those vegetative state patients/unresponsive wakefulness syndrome (VS/UWS) who will recover usually evolve into an MCS (consciousness recovery), then possibly present a functional recovery,

Table 2.1 Clinical evolution at 3, 6, and 12 months post-onset for vegetative state/unresponsive wakefulness syndrome (*VS/UWS*) patients and for minimally conscious state (*MCS*) patients (in %)

Diagnosis 1 month post-injury	3 months (%)	6 months (%)	12 months (%)
VS-traumatic (*n* = 52)			
Dead	21	31	42
VS	56	33	21
MCS	21	23	14
Emergence from MCS	2	13	23
VS-non-traumatic (*n* = 64)			
Dead	30	52	70
VS	64	38	20
MCS	6	9	8
Emergence from MCS	0	1	2
MCS-traumatic (*n* = 35)			
Dead	6	14	23
VS	17	6	0
MCS	60	40	29
Emergence from MCS	17	40	48
MCS-non-traumatic (*n* = 49)			
Dead	14	18	33
VS	20	4	2
MCS	64	61	39
Emergence from MCS	2	17	26

reflecting the emergence from MCS and this with or without physical, psychological, or neuropsychological disorders [9] (Fig. 2.1).

Several studies attempted to quantify the mortality rate and the degree of recovery of patients with disorders of consciousness (Tables 2.2, 2.3, and 2.4). Although these studies are informative, they have limitations, and for several reasons they cannot guide healthcare professionals and families in making treatment decisions: (1) most of these studies only included VS/UWS patients and very few studied MCS patients; (2) the majority were conducted before the establishment of MCS criteria (published in 2002) and, therefore, considered VS/UWS and MCS as a single condition, which is not correct; (3) the inclusion criteria were poorly defined; and finally (4) the number of patients included in these studies was limited, making findings difficult to generalize.

Recently, the Belgian Federal Ministry of Public Health launched a project on medical attitudes toward patients suffering from altered state of consciousness [11].

During the past 6 years, medical history, clinical, and epidemiological data were collected in 15 Belgian neurorehabilitation expertise centers [11]. These data allowed us to improve our knowledge of patients with altered state of consciousness – survival and recovery. In order to determine patients' consciousness state and to establish a reliable diagnosis, the Coma Recovery Scale-Revised (CRS-R) [12] was performed after 1, 3, 6, and 12 months post-injury. The prognosis was considered according to

Table 2.2 Mortality and recovery rates of traumatic vegetative state/unresponsive wakefulness syndrome patients

Authors	*N*	Duration post-onset	Follow-up	Results
Higashi et al. [8, 17]	38	3 months	1–5 years	3-year cumulative mortality rate: 55%, 5-year: 66%
Bricolo et al. [14]	135	2 weeks	1 year	30% dead, 8% VS/UWS, 31% severe disability, 18% moderate recovery, 13% good recovery. Age at onset influences patients' prognosis: mortality rate (16% for patients <20 years; 78% for patients >60 years) and good recovery (43%<20 years and 0%>60 years)
Braakman et al. [15]	140	1 month	1 year	51% dead, 11% VS/UWS, 26% severe disability, 10% moderate disability or recovery, 2% unknown (dead: 30% of after 3 months, 40% after 6 months). Duration of unconsciousness was negatively correlated with the functional recovery. No patients over 40 years showed any recovery allowing him to living independently
Sazbon [18]	55	1 month	1 year	51% recovery of consciousness
Sazbon and Groswasser [5]	134	1 month	1 year	54% recovery of consciousness, 46% VS/UWS
Sazbon and Groswasser [16]	134	1 month	1 year	3, 6, and 12-month cumulative mortality rate: 7%, 19%, and 32%
				5-year cumulative mortality rate: 68%
Multi-Society Task Force [10]	434	1 month	1 year	33% dead, 15% VS/UWS, 52% recovery of consciousness: 28% severe disability, 17% moderate disability, 7% good recovery
Danze et al. [19]	522	1 month	1 year	19% dead, 20% VS/UWS, 61% recovery of consciousness: 47% severe disability, 12% moderate disability, 2% good recovery. Mortality rate was positively correlated with the patient's age
Dubroja et al. [20]	19	1 month	2 years	68% recovery of consciousness (58% after 1 year, 5% after 2 years): 58% moderate disability, 42% severe disability
Giacino and Kalmar [21]	30	11±5 weeks	1 year	10% dead, 60% extremely severe disability or VS/UWS, 30% moderate to severe disability, 0% partial or good recovery
Estraneo et al. [22]	18	11 months	28±12 months	39% dead, 17% VS/UWS, 44% recovery of consciousness and functional recovery (17% MCS)

Table 2.3 Mortality and recovery rates of non-traumatic vegetative state patients

Authors	*N*	Etiology	Duration since onset	Follow-up	Results
Levy et al. [25]	25	Non-traumatic	1 month	1 year	72% dead, 8% intelligible words but no command following, 12% visual pursuit or localization to sounds. None of the patients can live independently
Sazbon [18]	118	Non-traumatic	1 month	1 year	21% recovery of consciousness
Sazbon et al. [24]	100	Anoxic	1 month	1–5 years	1 year post-onset: 46% dead, 20% conscious (13% after 3 months, 20% after 6 months, 17% tetraparetic, 19% cognitive disability, 15% dysphasic and 13% psychological disability), 33% unconscious, 1% unknown 5 years post-onset: 68% dead, 20% conscious, 7% unconscious, 5% unknown Cumulative mortality rate: 15% at 3 months, 31% at 6 months After 5 months of VS/UWS, no recovery of consciousness. Age at onset influences motor status and independence degree in daily living but not the cognitive status or psychological disorders
Multi-Society Task Force [10]	169	Non-traumatic	1 month	1 year	53% dead, 32% VS/UWS, 11% severe disability, 3% moderate disability, 1% good recovery
Giacino and Kalmar [21]	34	Non-traumatic	11 ± 5 weeks	1 year	7% dead, 87% extremely severe disability or VS/UWS, 6% severe to moderate disability, 0% partial or total recovery
Estraneo et al. [22]	50	Hemorragic	12 months	26 ± 13 months	4% dead, 50% VS/UWS, 6% recovery of consciousness (6% MCS)
		Anoxic	9 months	23 ± 12 months	43% dead, 36% VS/UWS, 20% recovery of consciousness and functional recovery (7% MCS)

Table 2.4 Mortality and recovery rates of minimally conscious state patients

Authors	*N*	Etiology	Diagnostic	Duration post-onset	Follow-up	Results
Grosswasser and Sazbon [27]	72	Traumatic	MCS	1 month to 1 year	More than 2 years	49% independent, 9% partially independent, 32% dependant for daily activities, 40% no work, 49% sheltered workshops, 11% job similar to the one practiced before the accident
Sazbon and Groswasser [28]	72	Traumatic	MCS	1 month to 1 year	1 year	VS/UWS < 2 months ($n = 38$): <50% independent for daily living activities, <90% cognitive deficit VS/UWS > 6 months ($n = 4$): 0% independent for daily living activities, 100% cognitive deficits
Giacino and Kalmar [21]	30	Traumatic	MCS	9 ± 5 weeks	1 year	0% dead, 17% extremely severe disability or VS/UWS, 60% severe to moderate disability, 3% partial or good recovery
	10	Non-traumatic				20% dead, 30% extremely severe disability or VS/UWS, 50% severe to moderate disability, 0% total recovery
Lammi et al. [29]	18	Traumatic	MCS	1 month	2–5 years	10% dead, 20% extremely severe disability or VS/UWS, 55% severe to moderate disability, 15% partial or good recovery
Katz et al. [30]	36	Traumatic and Non-traumatic	VS/UWS (11) (3 non-traumatic) MCS (25) (11 non-traumatic)	1 month	1–4 years	Last evaluation showed that 72% emerged from the MCS. Time to emerge was more important for VS/UWS patients as compared to MCS patients. 73% of the VS/UWS patients evolved to a MCS (87% traumatic, 33% non-traumatic), 72% of the MCS patients emerged after 9 weeks (mean). Emergence from the MCS was more frequent for MCS patients as compared to VS/UWS patients. Last evaluation showed that 27% of the patients present partial disability, 41% moderate disability, 32% severe to extremely severe disability
Luauté et al. [26]	39	Traumatic and Non-traumatic	MCS	1 year	5 years	36% dead, 33% severe disability, 23% MCS. Information no available for three patients

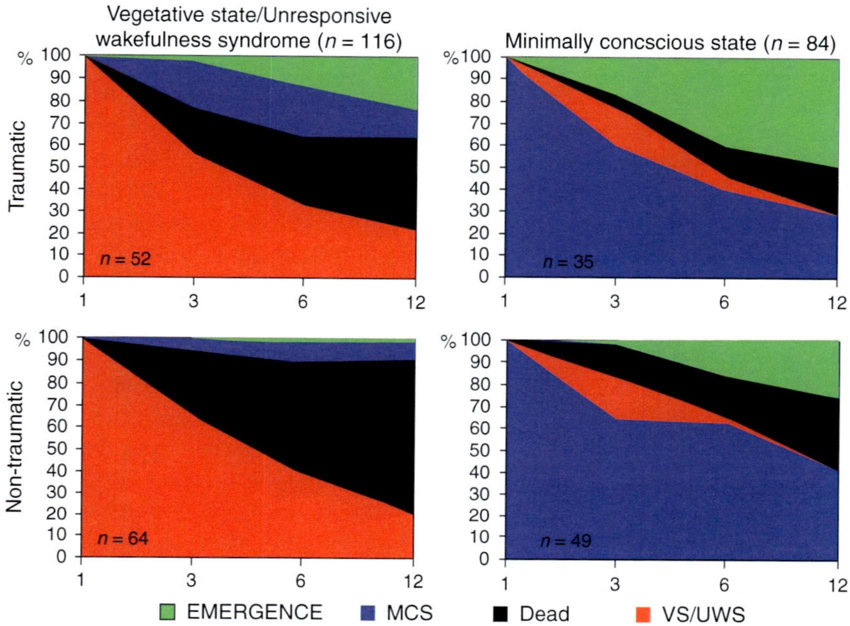

Fig. 2.2 Clinical evolution at 3, 6, and 12 months (abscissa) post-onset for vegetative state (*VS/UWS*) patients and for minimally conscious state (*MCS*) patients. In *red*: VS/UWS patients; in *blue*: MCS; in *black*: dead patients; in *green*: emergence from MCS

the three dimensions mentioned above – survival/mortality, recovery of consciousness (MCS), and functional recovery (emergence from MCS). Our study is one of the few to have established a clear distinction between recovery of consciousness and functional recovery. This distinction allowed us to identify (1) VS/UWS patients (at 1 month post-injury) who progressed to MCS 1 year after the insult (recovery of consciousness); (2) VS/UWS patients that emerged from MCS (functional recovery); and finally (3) MCS patients (1 month after the accident) who emerged from this state (functional recovery) 1 year later. Two hundred patients were included in our study: 116 patients were diagnosed VS/UWS and 84 patients were diagnosed MCS 1 month after injury. Among VS/UWS patients, 52 were traumatic cases (traffic accident, work accident, fall, violence, etc.) and 64 were Non-traumatic cases (anoxia, stroke, intoxication, infection, brain tumor, etc.). Of the 84 MCS patients, etiology was traumatic in 35 and non-traumatic in 49 (Table 2.1, Fig. 2.2). Compared to previous findings, our study presents some important strengths: (1) it includes a large number of patients, (2) it properly assigns a standardized diagnosis to patients, (3) it differentiates the prognosis for VS/UWS and MCS patients using etiology – traumatic versus Non-traumatic – as adjustment factor.

Mortality Rate

In our study, we found that in traumatic VS/UWS patients, 1 year post-onset mortality rate was 42% [13]. These results are in line with previous studies showing VS/UWS patients mortality rates ranging from 30% to 50% [10, 14–16]. In 1980, Bricolo and colleagues studied the prognosis of 135 patients who stayed in a "nonresponsive state" at least 2 weeks post-onset and had a mortality rate of 30% after 1 year [14]. Braakman and colleagues followed, for 1 year, 140 VS/UWS patients and observed a mortality rate of 51% [15]. Finally, the Multi-Society Task Force studied 434 patients and reported a mortality rate of 33% [10] (Table 2.2).

Regarding Non-traumatic VS/UWS patients' mortality rate, previous studies showed rates ranging from 50% to 70%. In 1978, Levy and colleagues reported a mortality rate of 70% at 1-year post-injury ($n=25$) [23] – this is in line with our observation (mortality rate of 70%; $n=64$). The Multi-Society Task Force [10], Estraneo and colleagues [22], and Sazbon and colleagues [24] report mortality rates of 53% ($n=169$), 43% ($n=32$), and 46% ($n=100$), respectively. These observed differences could be explained by the limited number of patients included in these studies [22, 23] and by the choice of inclusion criteria (duration of the non-response state ranging from 1 month [23] to 1 year [22] (post-onset)) (Table 2.3). Finally, like in previous studies, our study revealed a higher mortality rate in non-traumatic VS/UWS patients as compared to traumatic VS/UWS patients [5, 8, 10, 17, 22, 24, 26].

To date, only a few studies have examined MCS patients' mortality rates (Table 2.4), and most of them presented some limitations. Indeed, due to the low number of observations [21, 29] and the lack of information concerning patients' etiology [26], it is challenging to generalize findings from the literature. In 2005, Lammi and colleagues studied 18 traumatic MCS patients and observed, 1 year post-injury, a 10% mortality rate [29]. In the works of Giacino and Kalmar, mortality rates were 20% for Non-traumatic MCS patients ($n=10$), and there were no death in MCS traumatic patients ($n=30$) [21]. Finally, a recent study published by Luauté and collaborators [26] showed a mortality rate of 36%; however, no distinction was made for etiologies ($n=36$). In our recent study, we showed a 23% mortality rate in traumatic MCS patients ($n=35$) and 33% in non-traumatic patients ($n=49$) [13]. These findings expand the knowledge on the prognosis of patients suffering from disorders of consciousness by providing information on MCS patients' mortality rate and are in line with previous studies showing prognosis differences according to the etiology of VS/UWS or MCS [10, 21].

Recovery of Consciousness and Functional Recovery

VS/UWS Patients

In VS/UWS patients, consciousness recovery and functional recovery can be considered as a single category. We will then use the general term "recovery." In the literature, recovery rates range from 40% to 60% for traumatic VS/UWS patients.

In our study, we found a recovery rate of 37% 1 year post-onset ($n=52$) [13]. Results obtained by Braakman and colleagues ($n=140$) [31] and Estraneo and colleagues ($n=18$) [22] are in line with our study, showing recovery rates of 36% and 44%, respectively. Sazbon and colleagues showed a rate of 51% ($n=55$) [18], the Multi-Society Task Force a rate of 52% ($n=434$) [10], Giacino and Kalmar of 56% ($n=30$) [21], Dubroja and colleagues [20] of 58% ($n=19$), and Bricolo and colleagues [14] observed a recovery rate of 62% ($n=135$). The variability of these results could be explained by the patients' inclusion criteria and by the definition of "recovery" used by the different authors. Concerning non-traumatic VS/UWS patients, our results are in line with previous studies showing recovery rate ranging from 0% to 21%, 1 year post-onset [10, 18, 23, 24, 32].

With regard to the recovery of consciousness in VS/UWS patients (VS/UWS patients evolving to MCS), we observed that 14% of traumatic patients ($n=52$) and 8% of non-traumatic patients ($n=64$) recovered consciousness [13]. Our results are in line with those of Estraneo and colleagues [22] who followed for 2 years 18 traumatic VS/UWS patients and 32 non-traumatic VS/UWS patients. They noted a consciousness recovery rate of 17% for traumatic patients and 7% for non-traumatic patients. If one focuses on the functional recovery in VS/UWS patients (patients emerging from MCS), findings from previous studies are difficult to compare since each study assessed functional recovery with different criteria and/or scales. Some studies estimated recovery using the Glasgow Outcome Scale [33] while others used the Disability Rating Scale [34]. The Glasgow Outcome Scale includes five categories. A score of 5 corresponds to a good recovery (independent patients with or without neurological deficit), a score of 4 is given to patients with moderate disability (independent patient with moderate neurological and/or intellectual deficit), a score of 3 corresponds to severe disability (conscious patient but totally dependent in daily living activities), a score of 2 characterizes VS/UWS patients, and finally a score of 1 is assigned to dead patients. The Disability Rating Scale assesses the level of functioning of patients by scoring their level of ability. A total score of 30 is assigned to dead patients, a score between 25 and 29 correspond to patients who are *extremely vegetative*, 22–24 for VS/UWS patients, 17–21 characterized patients with extreme severe deficits, 12–16 characterized patients with severe deficits, 7–11 moderate to severe deficits, 4–6 moderate deficits, 2–3 partial or light deficits, and finally a score of 0 is given to patients with no deficit. It has to be noted that with these two scales, MCS patients and patients who emerged from MCS would be classified in the same category; they would obtain the same score of 3 with the Glasgow Outcome Scale and a score between 17 and 21 with the Disability Rating Scale. This means that patients with different level of functional recovery would receive the same scoring and be classified in a single category. This obviously raises several difficulties in the quantification, interpretation, and generalization of results reported by studies using such assessment tools.

In our research, we report a functional recovery rate – emergence from MCS 1 year after initial brain injury – of 23% in traumatic patients who were VS/UWS 1 month after onset [13]. A previous study on traumatic VS/UWS patients outcome, from Bricolo and collaborators [14], reports 1 year posttrauma severe disability in 31%, moderate recovery in 18%, and good recovery in 13% ($n=135$) of observed patients.

Braakman and colleagues noted 26% of severe disability and 10% of moderate or complete recovery (defined as patients being able to live independently) 1 year post-onset ($n=140$). In 1994, out of 522 patients, Danze and colleagues reported that 14% of patients recovered cognitive and motor capacities allowing them to live independently [19]. Giacino and Kalmar [21] reported a recovery rate of 30% ($n=30$), and finally the Multi-Society Task Force found that 28% of studied patients presented severe deficits, 17% moderate deficits, and 7% good recovery 1 year post-onset ($n=434$) [10]. Although these results are difficult to generalize, we can estimate that functional recovery rate in traumatic VS/UWS patients ranges between 10% and 30%.

It is, however, important to mention that the rate of patients living independently is very limited – ranges between 0% and 14%. Our study showed that non-traumatic VS/UWS patients presented a functional recovery rate as low as 2% 1 year after the onset.

Similarly, Levy and colleagues [23] observed that, out of their 25 studied patients, no patient recovered a functional status that would allow independent living. The Multi-Society Task Force showed that, out of the 169 patients studied, 3% presented moderate deficits and only 1% had a good recovery [10]. One should note that late recovery (more than a year post-injury) remains possible and occurs more frequently for traumatic patients [8, 10, 35–37].

MCS Patients

Our study showed that the rate of traumatic MCS patients emerging from MCS – functional recovery – is about 48%. Giacino and Kalmar [21] assessed the degree of recovery in 30 MCS patients using the Disability Rating Scale, and reported 23% of complete or partial recovery and 60% of poor to moderate recovery. Grosswasser and Sazbon [27] assessed functional recovery in 72 traumatic MCS patients (out of a group of 134 patients) and found that 49% of them could live independently, while 19% were partly dependent and 32% remained dependent in daily activities. Regarding the patients' occupational status, 11% found an employment similar to the employment they had before the accident, 49% of the patients are employed in sheltered workshops, and 40% were unable to reenter in the world of work.

In 2005, Lammi and colleagues [29] studied the recovery of 18 traumatic MCS patients and showed that 55% of them presented moderate to severe deficits whereas 15% presented good recovery or minor deficits.

For non-traumatic MCS patients, our study showed that functional recovery occurred in 26% of the cases. Only one study looked at the functional recovery rate of non-traumatic MCS patients and showed moderate to severe deficits in 50% of the cases while no good recovery was observed ($n=10$) [21]. However, this study included only a few numbers of patients making results impossible to interpret. We also found that functional recovery rate (emergence from MCS – functional communication and/or functional objects use) was higher for MCS patients as compared to VS/UWS patients, regardless of etiology. Indeed, 23% of the traumatic VS/UWS patients as compared to 48% of MCS patients recovered a functional communication and/or a functional use of objects 1 year post-onset.

Our results are similar for non-traumatic patients, 2% of functional recovery for VS/UWS patients and 26% for MCS patients – in line with previous studies evaluating the functional recovery of VS/UWS and MCS patients [21, 26, 30].

Note also that a study including 72 traumatic patients showed that the duration of unconsciousness in the acute stage influenced the prognosis 1 year post-onset. Patients who did not emerge from the VS/UWS within 6 months had a worse disability level than those who showed signs of consciousness during this period [28].

Finally, other studies have demonstrated the importance of the age at the time of the accident. Children between 5- and 6-years old are more likely to present favorable prognosis than adults [8, 10, 15, 38–41]. Patients older than 40 years have less chance to present favorable prognosis than young patients [10, 27, 42]. However, these results need to be confirmed by further studies based on a larger number of patients, with clearly defined inclusion criteria, and with a better distinction between degrees of recovery (MCS or emergence from MCS).

Conclusion

Data from our study showed that mortality rate in VS/UWS patients was higher than in MCS patients, regardless of the etiology. In addition, patients with non-traumatic brain injury have a higher mortality rate than traumatic patients. The same observations were noted regarding the patients' degree of functional recovery. We observed that, whatever the etiology, MCS patients have a better functional recovery than VS/UWS patients. Similarly, traumatic patients were more likely to present functional recovery than patients with a non-traumatic etiology [13].

In patients with altered state of consciousness, a reliable prognosis is a fundamental aspect of the care, from the intensive care units to the long-term life institution. Surgical, medical, or ethical decisions will depend upon this information. While it is legitimate to set up a high medical and therapeutic cares for patients with a good prognosis, it may not be desirable for most medical and paramedical teams to promote such treatments when the predictable prognosis is bad. Scientific advances allow a better understanding of the mortality rate and the degree of recovery in VS/UWS and MCS patients; however, medical staff and the family should be cautious regarding ethical decisions. We demonstrated that the MCS entity is different from the VS/UMS, the outcome of MCS patients being significantly better than that of VS/UWS patients. In addition, we know that the etiology of brain injury influences patients' prognosis. Traumatic patients are more likely to recover functional communication than non-traumatic patients. However, further studies still need be done to better characterize the functional recovery of patients who emerged from MCS and to better quantify the cognitive impairments of these patients.

References

1. Teasdale G, Jennett B. Assessment of coma and impaired consciousness. A practical scale. Lancet. 1974;2:81–4.
2. Boveroux P, Kirsch M, Boly M, et al. Neurologic prognosis assessment in postanoxic encephalopathy. Reanimation. 2008;17:613–7.
3. Kirsch M, Boveroux P, Massion P, et al. Comment prédire l'évolution du coma post-anoxique ? Rev Med Liege. 2008;63:263–8.
4. Wijdicks EF, Hijdra A, Young GB, et al. Practice parameter: prediction of outcome in comatose survivors after cardiopulmonary resuscitation (an evidence-based review): report of the Quality Standards Subcommittee of the American Academy of Neurology. Neurology. 2006;67:203–10.
5. Sazbon L, Groswasser Z. Outcome in 134 patients with prolonged posttraumatic unawareness. Part 1: parameters determining late recovery of consciousness. J Neurosurg. 1990;72:75–80.
6. Jennett B, Teasdale G, Braakman R, et al. Predicting outcome in individual patients after severe head injury. Lancet. 1976;1:1031–4.
7. The Multi-Society Task Force on PVS. Medical aspects of the persistent vegetative state (1). N Engl J Med. 1994;330:1499–508.
8. Higashi K, Sakata Y, Hatano M, et al. Epidemiological studies on patients with a persistent vegetative state. J Neurol Neurosurg Psychiatry. 1977;40:876–85.
9. Giacino JT, Ashwal S, Childs N, et al. The minimally conscious state: definition and diagnostic criteria. Neurology. 2002;58:349–53.
10. The Multi-Society Task Force on PVS. Medical aspects of the persistent vegetative state (2). N Engl J Med. 1994;330:1572–9.
11. Demotte R. Politique de la santé à mener à l'égard des patients en état végétatif persistant ou en état pauci-relationnel. Moniteur Belge 2004:69334–40.
12. Giacino JT, Kalmar K, Whyte J. The JFK coma recovery scale-revised: measurement characteristics and diagnostic utility. Arch Phys Med Rehabil. 2004;85:2020–9.
13. Bruno MA, Gosseries O, Vanhaudenhuyse A, et al. État végétatif et état de conscience minimale: un devenir pire que la mort ? In: Puybasset L, editor. Enjeux éthiques en réanimation. Paris: Springer; 2010. p. 119–28.
14. Bricolo A, Turazzi S, Feriotti G. Prolonged posttraumatic unconsciousness: therapeutic assets and liabilities. J Neurosurg. 1980;52:625–34.
15. Braakman R, Jennett WB, Minderhoud JM. Prognosis of the posttraumatic vegetative state. Acta Neurochir. 1988;95:49–52.
16. Sazbon L, Groswasser Z. Medical complications and mortality of patients in the postcomatose unawareness (PC-U) state. Acta Neurochir (Wien). 1991;112:110–2.
17. Higashi K, Hatano M, Abiko S, et al. Five-year follow-up study of patients with persistent vegetative state. J Neurol Neurosurg Psychiatry. 1981;44:552–4.
18. Sazbon L. Prolonged coma. Prog Clin Neurosci. 1985;2:65–81.
19. Danze F, Veys B, Lebrun T, et al. Prognostic factors of post-traumatic vegetative states: 522 cases. Neurochirurgie. 1994;40:348–57. discussion 357–348.
20. Dubroja I, Valent S, Miklic P, Kesak D. Outcome of post-traumatic unawareness persisting for more than a month. J Neurol Neurosurg Psychiatry. 1995;58:465–6.
21. Giacino JT, Kalmar K. The vegetative and minimally conscious states: a comparison of clinical features and functional outcome. J Head Trauma Rehabil. 1997;12:36–51.
22. Estraneo A, Moretta P, Loreto V, et al. Late recovery after traumatic, anoxic, or hemorrhagic long-lasting vegetative state. Neurology. 2010;75:239–45.
23. Levy DE, Knill-Jones RP, Plum F. The vegetative state and its prognosis following nontraumatic coma. Ann N Y Acad Sci. 1978;315:293–306.
24. Sazbon L, Zagreba F, Ronen J, et al. Course and outcome of patients in vegetative state of nontraumatic aetiology. J Neurol Neurosurg Psychiatry. 1993;56:407–9.
25. Levy DE. Coma after cardiac arrest–how Much care is enough? [editorial]. West J Med. 1987;147:191–3.

26. Luaute J, Maucort-Boulch D, Tell L, et al. Long-term outcomes of chronic minimally conscious and vegetative states. Neurology. 2010;75:246–52.
27. Groswasser Z, Sazbon L. Outcome in 134 patients with prolonged posttraumatic unawareness. Part 2: functional outcome of 72 patients recovering consciousness. J Neurosurg. 1990;72:81–4.
28. Sazbon L, Groswasser Z. Time-related sequelae of TBI in patients with prolonged post-comatose unawareness (PC-U) state. Brain Inj. 1991;5:3–8.
29. Lammi MH, Smith VH, Tate RL, Taylor CM. The minimally conscious state and recovery potential: a follow-up study 2 to 5 years after traumatic brain injury. Arch Phys Med Rehabil. 2005;86:746–54.
30. Katz DI, Polyak M, Coughlan D, et al. Natural history of recovery from brain injury after prolonged disorders of consciousness: outcome of patients admitted to inpatient rehabilitation with 1–4 year follow-up. Prog Brain Res. 2009;177:73–88.
31. Braakman R, Gelpke GJ, Habbema JD, et al. Systematic selection of prognostic features in patients with severe head injury. Neurosurgery. 1980;6:362–70.
32. Giacino JT. The vegetative and minimally conscious states: consensus-based criteria for establishing diagnosis and prognosis. NeuroRehabilitation. 2004;19:293–8.
33. Jennett B, Bond M. Assessment of outcome after severe brain damage. Lancet. 1975;1:480–4.
34. Rappaport M, Hall KM, Hopkins K, et al. Disability rating scale for severe head trauma: coma to community. Arch Phys Med Rehabil. 1982;63:118–23.
35. Avesani R, Gambini MG, Albertini G. The vegetative state: a report of two cases with a long-term follow-up. Brain Inj. 2006;20:333–8.
36. Childs NL, Mercer WN. Late improvement in consciousness after post-traumatic vegetative state. N Engl J Med. 1996;334:24–5.
37. Voss HU, Uluc AM, Dyke JP, et al. Possible axonal regrowth in late recovery from the minimally conscious state. J Clin Invest. 2006;116:2005–11.
38. Kriel RL, Krach LE, Jones-Saete C. Outcome of children with prolonged unconsciousness and vegetative states. Pediatr Neurol. 1993;9:362–8.
39. Johnston RB, Mellits ED. Pediatric coma: prognosis and outcome. Dev Med Child Neurol. 1980;22:3–12.
40. Bruce DA, Schut L, Bruno LA, et al. Outcome following severe head injuries in children. J Neurosurg. 1978;48:679–88.
41. Ashwal S. The persistent vegetative state in children. Adv Pediatr. 1994;41:195–222.
42. Strauss DJ, Shavelle RM, Ashwal S. Life expectancy and median survival time in the permanent vegetative state. Pediatr Neurol. 1999;21:626–31.

Chapter 3
Functional Imaging and Impaired Consciousness

Audrey Vanhaudenhuyse, Melanie Boly, Marie-Aurélie Bruno, Olivia Gosseries, Athena Demertzi, Murielle Kirsch, Jean-Flory Luaba Tshibanda, Marie Thonnard, Vanessa Charland-Verville, Camille Chatelle, Aurore Thibaut, Steven Laureys, and Andrea Soddu

A. Vanhaudenhuyse, Ph.D. (✉) • M.-A. Bruno, Ph.D. • A. Demertzi, M.Sc.
V. Charland-Verville, M.Sc. • S. Laureys, M.D., Ph.D. • M. Thonnard, M.Sc.
Coma Science Group, Cyclotron Research Center, University of Liège,
Allée du 6 Août, Sart Tilman B30, 4000 Liège, Belgium

Department of Neurology, University Hospital of Liège, Liège, Belgium
e-mail: avanhaudenhuyse@ulg.ac.be; ma.bruno@ulg.ac.be; a.demertzi@ulg.ac.be; v.charland@student.ulg.ac.be; steven.laureys@ulg.ac.be; marie.thonnard@ulg.ac.be

M. Boly, M.D., Ph.D. • A. Soddu, Ph.D.
Coma Science Group, Cyclotron Research Center, University of Liège,
Allée du 6 Août, Sart Tilman B30, 4000 Liège, Belgium
e-mail: mboly@ulg.ac.be; andrea.soddu@ulg.ac.be

O. Gosseries, M.Sc. • C. Chatelle • A. Thibaut
Coma Science Group, Cyclotron Research Center, University of Liège,
Allée du 6 Août, Sart Tilman B30, 4000 Liège, Belgium

Department of Neurology, University Hospital of Liège, Liège, Belgium

National Fund for Scientific Research, Liège, Belgium
e-mail: ogosseries@doct.ulg.ac.be

M. Kirsch, M.D.
Coma Science Group, Cyclotron Research Center, University of Liège,
Allée du 6 Août, Sart Tilman B30, 4000 Liège, Belgium

Department of Anesthesiology, University Hospital of Liège, Sart Tilman, 4000 Liège, Belgium
e-mail: murielle.kirsch@chu.ulg.ac.be

J.-F.L. Tshibanda, M.D.
Coma Science Group, Cyclotron Research Center, University of Liège,
Allée du 6 Août, Sart Tilman B30, 4000 Liège, Belgium

Department of Radiology, University Hospital of Liège, Sart Tilman, 4000 Liège, Belgium
e-mail: l.tshibanda@chu.ulg.ac.be

C. Schnakers, S. Laureys (eds.), *Coma and Disorders of Consciousness*,
DOI 10.1007/978-1-4471-2440-5_3, © Springer-Verlag London 2012

Introduction

Differentiating a voluntary from a reflexive behavior in patients unable to communicate remains a big challenge. Currently, 40% of patients with disorders of consciousness are misdiagnosed as being in vegetative state when assessed with nonstandardized scales [1]. Along with more traditional electroencephalographic techniques, magnetic resonance imaging (MRI) and positron emission tomography (PET) offer today the opportunity to study the neural correlates of consciousness in patients with altered states of consciousness as compared to healthy subjects. While some methods are devoted to detecting cortical responses during sensory stimulation (tactile, auditory, visual, etc.), others propose to measure neural activity at rest or during "*active*" paradigms, requiring participation of the subject who have to perform mental imagery tasks. In this chapter, we propose a differentiated approach to study brain functions of patients in an altered state of consciousness, by combining multimodal assessment techniques such as PET and functional MRI (fMRI), to distinguish patients in a vegetative state (unconscious) from patients in a minimally conscious state (Fig. 3.1).

Brain Activity at Rest: Is There Any Implication for Consciousness?

Several studies using PET have shown a massive decrease in global cerebral metabolism for patients in vegetative state and coma, ranging from 40% to 50% (for a review, see [2]). However, patients recovering from a vegetative state do not show a

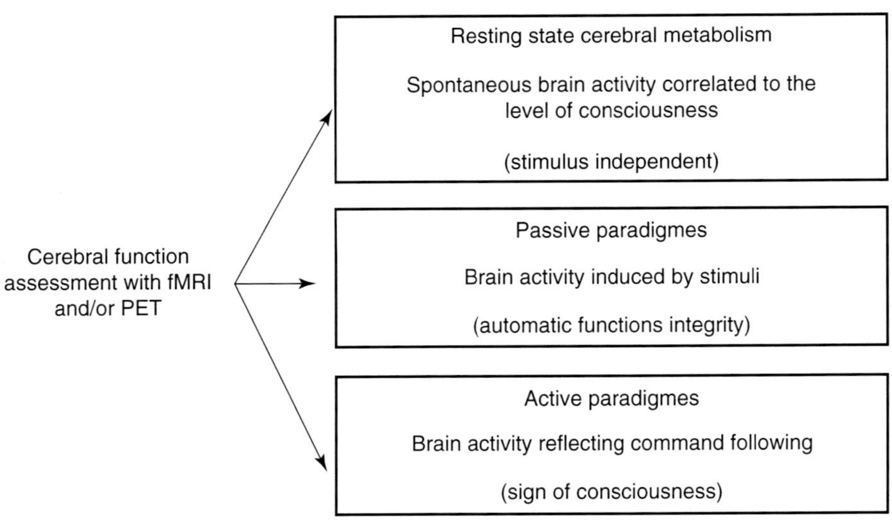

Fig. 3.1 Differentiated approach to study brain functions in patients with an altered state of consciousness combining multimodal assessment techniques such as positron emission tomography (*PET*) and functional magnetic resonance imaging (*fMRI*) (Adapted from [2])

systematic recovery of global brain metabolism to normal values [3]. Similarly, some healthy subjects demonstrate a metabolism comparable to what is observed in vegetative state patients [4]. Furthermore, vegetative state is characterized by a dysfunction of local rather than global cerebral areas, and specifically of the regions encompassing bilateral frontal, parieto-temporal, posterior parietal, mesiofrontal, posterior cingulate, and precuneal cortices [5, 6]. These brain areas are consistently more hypometabolic in vegetative state than in minimally conscious state patients [6], and are usually preserved in patients emerging from the minimally conscious state who recovered the ability to communicate [7]. Moreover, awareness seems related not exclusively to the activity in the frontoparietal network but, as importantly, to the functional connectivity within this network and the thalami. Indeed, long-range cortico-cortical and cortico-thalamo-cortical "*functional disconnections*" have been identified in the vegetative state [8]. The vegetative state seems also characterized by hypermetabolism in the reticular ascending system and a deficient functional connectivity between this system and the precuneus [9]. Finally, in a recent study measuring cerebral metabolism, we were able to demonstrate that the presence of visual fixation in nontraumatic brain-injured patients otherwise showing typical clinical characteristics of vegetative state was not accompanied by a different brain activity compared to patients in vegetative state showing no visual fixation [10]. Patients without visual fixation showed hypometabolism in the fronto-temporo-parietal cortex and thalami, similar to patients with visual fixation. No difference in recovery of consciousness could be identified between the two groups. These recent findings suggest that sustained visual fixation in nontraumatic disorders of consciousness should be considered carefully when giving a diagnosis of consciousness. In addition to the interest in measuring brain metabolism, an increasing attention is also drawn to spontaneous brain activity and its possible relevance for cognitive behavior [11]. Gusnard and Raichle [12] proposed the concept of default mode network after observing that most of the studies in PET and functional MRI (fMRI) reported a set of brain areas exhibiting task-induced deactivations, encompassing precuneus, posterior parietal lobe, and medial prefrontal cortex, which are more active at rest than when subjects were involved in attention-demanding cognitive tasks. These decreases in activity are considered as a reflection of suppression in information processing for the brain regions not involved in the task [13], and have a quite consistent spatial pattern [12]. If the exact function of the default mode network is still debated, some studies suggest that it could be involved in conscious perception processing. Moreover, the default mode network is known to be implicated in specific cognitive processes such as internal and stimuli independent thoughts [14, 15]. The study of the default mode network has a clinical interest in patients in an altered state of consciousness, since it allows the investigation of higher-order cognitive networks without requiring patients' active participation, particularly important in vegetative and minimally conscious patients. A recent work showed that no default mode network was detected in a brain death patient [2, 16] (Fig. 3.2), while vegetative state was characterized by a partial preservation of connectivity in the regions of the default mode network [16, 19]. Moreover, we demonstrated that there was a correlation between the level of connectivity within

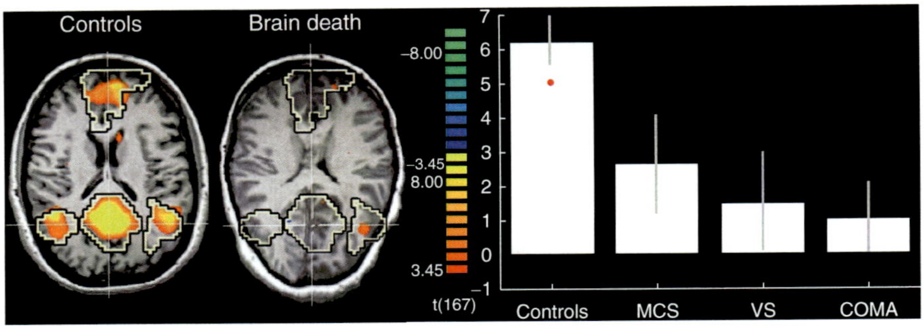

Fig. 3.2 Default mode network observed in healthy subjects (*yellow*). Brain death patients are characterized by a total absence of the network. The contours in *black* and *white* show the default mode network observed in a group of independent control subjects. *Chart* represents the nonlinear correlation between the level of consciousness of patients and the degree of connectivity of the precuneus with all the other regions of the default mode network (Adapted from [2, 51]). Locked-in syndrome: *red dot*, MCS minimally conscious state, VS vegetative state (Adapted from [2, 18])

the default mode network and the patients' level of consciousness (patients in coma, vegetative state, minimally conscious state and locked-in syndrome) [18] (Fig. 3.2). Specifically, the highest the drop in the level of awareness (coma, vegetative state), the most the degree of connectivity in the default mode network decreases. In addition, posterior cingulate cortex/precuneus was the region which better disentangles patients in vegetative and minimally consciousness state [18]. These results seem to sustain the hypothesis that the precuneus has a specific role in the architecture of the default mode network, as already indicated by functional [17] and structural [20] findings. All these results suggest that the default mode network is involved in the process of consciousness, completing previous studies, which show a partial preservation of the default mode network in light sleep [21] or in monkeys under general anesthesia [22]. These results also confirm recent studies showing a decrease in network connectivity in the default mode network in sedated healthy subjects [23] and deep sleep [24]. Finally, it is shared opinion that if the described findings seem very encouraging, most still need to be done to develop interpretable paradigms at the individual level, and therefore applicable for a clinical diagnosis of patients with severe brain injury, by developing techniques considering physiological and movement artifacts on the default mode network [25].

Brain Activation and External Stimuli: Conscious Perception?

Sensory perceptions (i.e., somatosensory, auditory, and visual) are related to conscious perception of stimulation. By definition, patients in vegetative state cannot consciously perceive these stimuli. However, we cannot exclude from behavioral observations that the stimuli presented are not perceived. In this context, various neuroimaging studies have investigated the brain activity observed during the presentation of different stimuli in disorders of consciousness patients. Several fMRI studies [26–29] have confirmed previous PET results, showing preserved brain activity in primary sensory cortex, but this activation is disconnected from all higher associative areas in patients in vegetative state both for auditory [30–32] and somatosensory [33, 34] stimulations. These studies also report that patients in minimally conscious state, compared to vegetative patients, have a much more distributed brain activity and cortico-cortical connectivity in response to stimuli, including nociceptive stimuli. These results emphasize the importance to adapt analgesic treatment in minimally conscious patients considering that their brain response during painful stimuli is very similar to the one observed in healthy subjects [33, 34]. In addition, for patients in minimally conscious state, auditory stimuli with emotional valence (i.e., cry of a baby, own name, and story narrated by a familiar voice) involve more areas than the ones observed in response to neutral stimuli in accordance to that observed in healthy individuals [35–37]. The activity of the anterior cingulate cortex has recently been demonstrated to correlate with the level of consciousness during the presentation of self-referential stimuli (patient's own name [38]). The highest the level of consciousness – in a minimally conscious state as compared to vegetative state patients – the greatest is the intensity of activation of the cingulate cortex. The fact that higher order areas are activated in minimally conscious state patients suggests that the content of our words may be relevant for the patient. Finally, some patients in vegetative state, even if exceptionally, may also show some activations in higher order areas in response to auditory [27, 32] or visual [32, 39] stimuli. The presence of unusual activity has been proposed as a possible prognostic marker for recovery of consciousness [40].

Active fMRI Paradigms: Help in the Diagnosis of Altered States of Consciousness?

Without a full understanding of brain mechanisms underlying consciousness, brain activation in patients similar to that observed in healthy subjects cannot be attributed to a conscious perception. The only conclusion one can draw is that these specific regions are able to process sensory stimuli [2]. Therefore, the question is how to distinguish an automatic brain response to a conscious perception. To overcome the problematic of disentangling automatic from conscious neuronal activity, Owen et al. [41] have proposed a different approach consisting in applying an active fMRI paradigm. A patient initially diagnosed as being in vegetative state was instructed to perform two mental imagery tasks, previously validated in a series of healthy volunteers [42]. In this study, when the patient was asked to "*imagine playing tennis*," an activation of the supplementary motor area was recorded; while the activation of parahippocampal gyri was observed when the patient was asked to "*imagine visiting her own house*." Such brain activations, similar to those observed in healthy volunteers, showed that the patient, on one hand, was able to understand instructions and, on the other hand, she was able to perform the imagery tasks. Note that these activations could be interpreted only as coming from an intentional participation of the patient. Indeed, even if the words "*tennis*" and "*home*" have already been reported as causing automatic brain activity – not aware – this activity is known to last only few milliseconds and appears only in areas related to word processing [43]. Brain activity lasted the entire period during which the patient was asked to perform the task (30 s) before resting, and was localized in areas known for their involvement in motor imagery tasks [42, 44, 45]. Owen et al. [45] conclude that such activations cannot be explained in terms of automatic responses. Interestingly, 6 months after this study, the patient showed behavioral signs of consciousness. Subsequently, this paradigm was applied in 54 patients in an altered state of consciousness (23 in a vegetative state, 31 in a minimally conscious state [46]). Among the studied patients, five (four initially diagnosed as being in a vegetative state and one in a minimally conscious state) showed classical brain activation observed for mental imagery tasks – in the supplementary motor area when patients were asked to perform the motor imagery task, and in the parahippocampal gyrus during the visuospatial task. This paradigm was then adapted into a yes/no answer communication system, allowing a patient with posttraumatic etiology to communicate without using the traditional communication channels (motor or language). This patient had received diagnosis of vegetative state 17 months after his traumatic accident. Five years after his injury, behavioral assessments showed reproducible signs of consciousness, reflecting a minimally conscious state. When inside the fMRI scanner, the patient was asked various biographical questions and instructed to answer "*yes*" by imagining playing tennis, or "*no*" by imagining visiting his home. The brain activity observed during the question sessions was similar to that observed in the training session in which the patient showed the ability to perform both imagery tasks [46], and was, respectively, translated in the yes/no answers for five out of the six questions (last question remained unanswered). The interpretation of these findings does not necessarily support the hypothesis that the patient was initially misdiagnosed. Indeed, it is plausible that the patient was in a vegetative state in the years before the fMRI scanning and that only gradually moved away from the vegetative state without, however, being able to behaviorally demonstrate his consciousness. Finally, 49 of the patients included in the latter study did not show any brain activation consistent with performing an imagery task. It is now difficult to say whether this absence is the result of a lack of sensitivity in the method, or whether it really reflects the inability or limitations in cognitive performance from the patients. Some patients could also be unconscious or sleeping during the fMRI session, as the arousal level can quickly fluctuate in these patients. For others, even in a minimally conscious state, the tasks could be cognitively too complex to be realized. Indeed, deficits in processes related to language comprehension, working memory, decision-making, or executive functions are all factors that can hinder a success of such tasks [47]. Conversely, one can conclude that patients' ability to perform these tasks demonstrates at least some preservation of cognitive processes. Voluntary brain modulation in fMRI was also recently demonstrated as a device of nonfunctional communication in a minimally conscious patient [48]. These studies show clearly a means to detect potentially existing dissociations between the behavior observed at the patients' bedside and their residual brain activity, reflecting preserved cognitive function [6, 49, 50]. This finding indicates that, in some patients, motor function can be so impaired that bedside assessments based on the presence or absence of a behavioral response may not reveal awareness, regardless of how thoroughly and carefully they are administered. These "*active*" paradigms must, therefore, be considered as an aid for diagnosis in patients with severe brain injury.

Conclusion

The difficulty in determining an accurate diagnosis and prognosis in patients surviving a coma has important ethical implications. Precise information based on scientific findings on the diagnosis and prognosis of the patient is essential to make the family understand and accept more easily medical decisions. The limits of behavioral assessments must encourage us to consider other biomarkers, which may be more objective for the detection of consciousness and may help clinicians in their evaluation. The various paradigms presented in this chapter demonstrate the value of neuroimaging techniques like PET or fMRI as diagnostic tools for patients in altered states of consciousness. Paradigms that study spontaneous activity may detect a residual level of consciousness without requiring the cooperation of patients. Active paradigms allow the detection of cognitive functions without involving language or motor responses. These paradigms give us the ability to differentiate vegetative from minimally conscious patients and can help to clarify the diagnosis of patients when behavioral assessments are ambiguous. PET allows identifying brain regions which present preserved metabolism, while fMRI allows identifying whether these regions are functionally interconnected or are more active during a task than at rest. By combining both techniques, more precise information regarding the functionality of cortical and subcortical regions could be obtained and potentially improve the diagnosis in patients with impaired consciousness. We also demonstrated the possibility of establishing a basic communication paradigm through two distinct (yes/no) imagery tasks inside the fMRI scanner. Unfortunately, this technique is impractical in everyday life but could definitely be used to allow patients expressing themselves on relevant issues such as their quality of life or decisions about their own care. Other methods, mostly based on electroencephalography, which may be adapted to everyday life, have already been used and are nowadays under development. By using these techniques, patients could express themselves on pain sensation and feelings. This would allow clinicians to adapt the treatment of patients, such as analgesic management for example. Finally, scientific advances in the area of disorders of consciousness and the possible clinical applications, makes possible to improve the diagnosis, refine the prognosis, and thus respond to ethical issues. However, neuroimaging techniques are still limited by artifacts induced, e.g., by the patient's movements inside the scanner, by artificial respiration, or by implanted ferromagnetic elements. Future work is, therefore, needed to reduce as much as possible these artifacts and new analyses need to be developed to eliminate residual contamination of the data.

References

1. Schnakers C, Vanhaudenhuyse A, Giacino J, et al. Diagnostic accuracy of the vegetative and minimally conscious state: clinical consensus versus standardized neurobehavioral assessment. BMC Neurol. 2009;9:35.
2. Bruno M, Soddu A, Demertzi A, et al. Disorders of consciousness: moving from passive to resting state and active paradigms. Cogn Neurosci. 2010;1(3):193–203.
3. Laureys S, Lemaire C, Maquet P, et al. Cerebral metabolism during vegetative state and after recovery to consciousness. J Neurol Neurosurg Psychiatry. 1999;67:121.
4. Laureys S. The neural correlate of (un) awareness: lessons from the vegetative state. Trends Cogn Sci. 2005;9:556–9.
5. Laureys S, Goldman S, Phillips C, et al. Impaired effective cortical connectivity in vegetative state. Neuroimage. 1999;9:377–82.
6. Laureys S, Owen AM, Schiff ND. Brain function in coma, vegetative state, and related disorders. Lancet Neurol. 2004;3:537–46.
7. Nakayama N, Okumura A, Shinoda J, et al. Relationship between regional cerebral metabolism and consciousness disturbance in traumatic diffuse brain injury without large focal lesions: an FDG-PET study with statistical parametric mapping analysis. J Neurol Neurosurg Psychiatry. 2006;77:856–62.
8. Laureys S, Faymonville ME, Luxen A, et al. Restoration of thalamocortical connectivity after recovery from persistent vegetative state. Lancet. 2000;355:1790–1.
9. Silva S, Alacoque X, Fourcade O, et al. Wakefulness and loss of awareness: brain and brainstem interaction in the vegetative state. Neurology. 2010;74:313–20.
10. Bruno MA, Vanhaudenhuyse A, Schnakers C, et al. Visual fixation in the vegetative state: an observational case series PET study. BMC Neurol. 2010;10:35.
11. Raichle ME. Neuroscience. The brain's dark energy. Science. 2006;314:1249–50.
12. Gusnard DA, Raichle ME. Searching for a baseline: functional imaging and the resting human brain. Nat Rev Neurosci. 2001;2:685–94.
13. Drevets WC, Burton H, Videen TO, et al. Blood flow changes in human somatosensory cortex during anticipated stimulation. Nature. 1995;373:249–52.
14. Mason MF, Norton MI, Van Horn JD, et al. Wandering minds: the default network and stimulus-independent thought. Science. 2007;315:393–5.
15. Vanhaudenhuyse A, Demertzi A, Schabus M, et al. Two distinct neuronal networks mediate the awareness of environment and of self. J Cogn Neurosci. 2011;23:570–8.
16. Boly M, Tshibanda L, Vanhaudenhuyse A, et al. Functional connectivity in the default network during resting state is preserved in a vegetative but not in a brain dead patient. Hum Brain Mapp. 2009;30:2393–400.
17. Fransson P, Marrelec G. The precuneus/posterior cingulate cortex plays a pivotal role in the default mode network: evidence from a partial correlation network analysis. Neuroimage. 2008;42:1178–84.
18. Vanhaudenhuyse A, Noirhomme Q, Tshibanda LJ, et al. Default network connectivity reflects the level of consciousness in non- communicative brain-damaged patients. Brain. 2010;133: 161–71.
19. Cauda F, Micon BM, Sacco K, et al. Disrupted intrinsic functional connectivity in the vegetative state. J Neurol Neurosurg Psychiatry. 2009;80:429–31.
20. Hagmann P, Cammoun L, Gigandet X, et al. Mapping the structural core of human cerebral cortex. PLoS Biol. 2008;6:e159.
21. Horovitz SG, Fukunaga M, de Zwart JA, et al. Low frequency BOLD fluctuations during resting wakefulness and light sleep: a simultaneous EEG-fMRI study. Hum Brain Mapp. 2008;29:671–82.
22. Vincent JL, Patel GH, Fox MD, et al. Intrinsic functional architecture in the anaesthetized monkey brain. Nature. 2007;447:83–6.

23. Greicius MD, Kiviniemi V, Tervonen O, et al. Persistent default-mode network connectivity during light sedation. Hum Brain Mapp. 2008;29:839–47.
24. Horovitz SG, Braun AR, Carr WS, et al. Decoupling of the brain's default mode network during deep sleep. Proc Natl Acad Sci USA. 2009;106:11376–81.
25. Soddu A, Vanhaudenhuyse A, Bahri MA, Bruno MA, Boly M, Demertzi A, Tshibanda JF, Phillips C, Stanziano M, Ovadia-Caro S, Nir Y, Maquet P, Papa M, Malach R, Laureys S, Noirhomme Q. Identifying the default-mode component in spatial IC analyses of patients with disorders of consciousness. Hum Brain Mapp. 2012;33:778–96.
26. Coleman MR, Rodd JM, Davis MH, et al. Do vegetative patients retain aspects of language comprehension? Evidence from fMRI. Brain. 2007;130:2494–507.
27. Di HB, Yu SM, Weng XC, et al. Cerebral response to patient's own name in the vegetative and minimally conscious states. Neurology. 2007;68:895–9.
28. Fernandez-Espejo D, Junque C, Vendrell P, et al. Cerebral response to speech in vegetative and minimally conscious states after traumatic brain injury. Brain Inj. 2008;22:882–90.
29. Moritz CH, Rowley HA, Haughton VM, et al. Functional MR imaging assessment of a non-responsive brain injured patient. Magn Reson Imaging. 2001;19:1129–32.
30. Boly M, Faymonville ME, Peigneux P, et al. Auditory processing in severely brain injured patients: differences between the minimally conscious state and the persistent vegetative state. Arch Neurol. 2004;61:233–8.
31. Laureys S, Faymonville ME, Degueldre C, et al. Auditory processing in the vegetative state. Brain. 2000;123(8):1589–601.
32. Owen AM, Menon DK, Johnsrude IS, et al. Detecting residual cognitive function in persistent vegetative state. Neurocase. 2002;8:394–403.
33. Boly M, Faymonville ME, Schnakers C, et al. Perception of pain in the minimally conscious state with PET activation: an observational study. Lancet Neurol. 2008;7(11):1013–20.
34. Laureys S, Faymonville ME, Peigneux P, et al. Cortical processing of noxious somatosensory stimuli in the persistent vegetative state. Neuroimage. 2002;17(2):732–41.
35. Laureys S, Perrin F, Faymonville ME, et al. Cerebral processing in the minimally conscious state. Neurology. 2004;63:916–8.
36. Bekinschtein T, Leiguarda R, Armony J, et al. Emotion processing in the minimally conscious state. J Neurol Neurosurg Psychiatry. 2004;75:788.
37. Schiff ND, Rodriguez-Moreno D, Kamal A, et al. FMRI reveals large-scale network activation in minimally conscious patients. Neurology. 2005;64:514–23.
38. Qin P, Di H, Liu Y, et al. Anterior cingulate activity and the self in disorders of consciousness. Hum Brain Mapp. 2010;31:1993–2002.
39. Menon DK, Owen AM, Williams EJ, et al. Cortical processing in persistent vegetative state. Lancet. 1998;352:200.
40. Di H, Boly M, Weng X, et al. Neuroimaging activation studies in the vegetative state: predictors of recovery? Clin Med. 2008;8:502–7.
41. Owen AM, Coleman MR, Boly M, et al. Detecting awareness in the vegetative state. Science. 2006;313:1402.
42. Boly M, Coleman MR, Davis MH, et al. When thoughts become action: an fMRI paradigm to study volitional brain activity in non- communicative brain injured patients. Neuroimage. 2007;36:979–92.
43. Hauk O, Johnsrude I, Pulvermuller F. Somatotopic representation of action words in human motor and premotor cortex. Neuron. 2004;41:301–7.
44. Weiskopf N, Mathiak K, Bock SW, et al. Principles of a brain- computer interface (BCI) based on real-time functional magnetic resonance imaging (fMRI). IEEE Trans Biomed Eng. 2004;51:966–70.
45. Owen A, Coleman M, Boly M, et al. Response to comments on detecting awareness in the vegetative state. Science. 2007;315:1221.
46. Monti MM, Vanhaudenhuyse A, Coleman MR, et al. Willful modulation of brain activity in disorders of consciousness. N Engl J Med. 2010;362:579–89.

47. Majerus S, Bruno MA, Schnakers C, et al. The problem of aphasia in the assessment of consciousness in brain-damaged patients. Prog Brain Res. 2009;177:49–61.
48. Bardin JC, Fins JJ, Katz DI, Hersh J, Heier LA, Tabelow K, Dyke JP, Ballon DJ, Schiff ND, Voss HU. Dissociations between behavioural and functional magnetic resonance imaging-based evaluations of cognitive function after brain injury. Brain. 2011;134:769–82.
49. Monti MM, Coleman MR, Owen AM. Neuroimaging and the vegetative state: resolving the behavioral assessment dilemma? Ann NY Acad Sci. 2009;1157:81–9.
50. Owen AM, Coleman MR. Functional neuroimaging of the vegetative state. Nat Rev Neurosci. 2008;9:235–43 Schnackers.
51. Tshibanda L, Vanhaudenhuyse A, Boly M, et al. Neuroimaging after coma. Neuroradiology. 2010;52:15–24.

Chapter 4
Multivariate Pattern Recognition Analysis: Brain Decoding

Jessica Schrouff and Christophe L.M. Phillips

Introduction

Two of the most fundamental questions in the field of neuroscience are how information is represented in different brain structures, and how this information evolves over time. Various tools, such as magnetic resonance imaging (MRI) and positron emission tomography (PET), have been developed over the last few decades to record brain activity and investigate these questions. In particular, functional MRI (fMRI) tracks changes of the blood oxygenation level-dependent (BOLD) signal, which is a good indicator of brain activity [1], with a spatial resolution of a few cubic millimeters and a typical temporal resolution in the order of 1 or 2 s.

Until recently, the methods used to analyze such data focused on characterizing the individual relationship between a cognitive or perceptual state and each image voxel, i.e., following a massively univariate statistical approach. A well-known univariate technique is statistical parametric mapping (SPM) [2]. SPM relies on the general linear model [3] to detect which voxels show a statistically significant response to the (combination of) experimental conditions of interest. However, there are limitations on what can be learned about the representation of information by examining voxels in a univariate fashion. For instance, spatially distributed sets of voxels considered as nonsignificant by a SPM analysis of one experimental condition might still carry information about the presence or absence of that condition. Furthermore, classic voxel-based analytic techniques are also mainly designed to perform group-wise comparisons and would, therefore, be unsuitable to evaluate the state of the disease of each individual.

On the other hand, multi-voxel pattern analyses (MVPA) [4–6] allow an increased sensitivity to detect the presence of a particular mental representation. These multivariate

J. Schrouff, M.Sc. (✉) • C.L.M. Phillips, Ph.D.
Cyclotron Research Center, University of Liège,
Allée du 6 Août, Sart Tilman B30, 4000 Liège, Belgium
e-mail: jschrouff@ulg.ac.be; c.phillips@ulg.ac.be

C. Schnakers, S. Laureys (eds.), *Coma and Disorders of Consciousness*,
DOI 10.1007/978-1-4471-2440-5_4, © Springer-Verlag London 2012

methods, also known as brain decoding or mind reading, attempt to link a particular cognitive, behavioral, perceptual, or medical state to specific patterns of voxels' activity. Application of these methods made it possible to decode the category of a seen object [7–9] or the orientation of a stripped pattern seen by the subject [10, 11] from the brain activation of the imaged subject. Advances in pattern-classification algorithms also allowed the decoding of less-controlled conditions such as memory retrieval tasks [12, 13]. Advanced mathematical tools are still under development to allow the classification of more complicated experimental data sets, such as examining the content of mind wandering or detecting the state of consciousness of a patient showing no response to a command.

Methodology

Multivariate pattern analysis derives from the fields of pattern recognition and machine learning, which are concerned with the automatic discovery of regularities in data. Those regularities then serve as the basis for the classification of new data. A classical example of pattern recognition is the automatic classification of handwritten digits (Fig. 4.1): each digit is represented by a grey scale image of 28×28 pixels and the goal is to build an algorithm capable of classifying each image into the correct category (i.e., 0, 1,..., 9). We, therefore, need to build an "algorithmic machine" that will take images as inputs and produce their corresponding digit as outputs. Due to the large variability in handwritings, this operation is not trivial and the use of machine learning is necessary. This means that the computer has to learn which pattern in the images corresponds to which digit. This learning is achieved by providing a "learning set," which is a set comprising both images (inputs) and corresponding digit (outputs). This is called "supervised learning." The machine can then build the required function using this learning set and finally assign outputs to new inputs. Similarly, instead of classifying data into discrete categories or outputs, a machine can be taught to regress out a continuous scalar from a series of inputs – after learning, the trained function can then predict the (continuous) outcome from

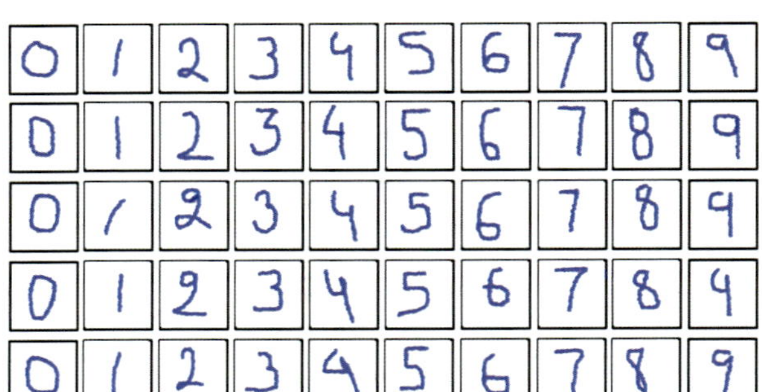

Fig. 4.1 Examples of handwritten digits. Each digit is discretized as a 28×28 pixel *grey scale image*. Practically speaking, more than those five examples of handwritten digits would be necessary to build an efficient classifier

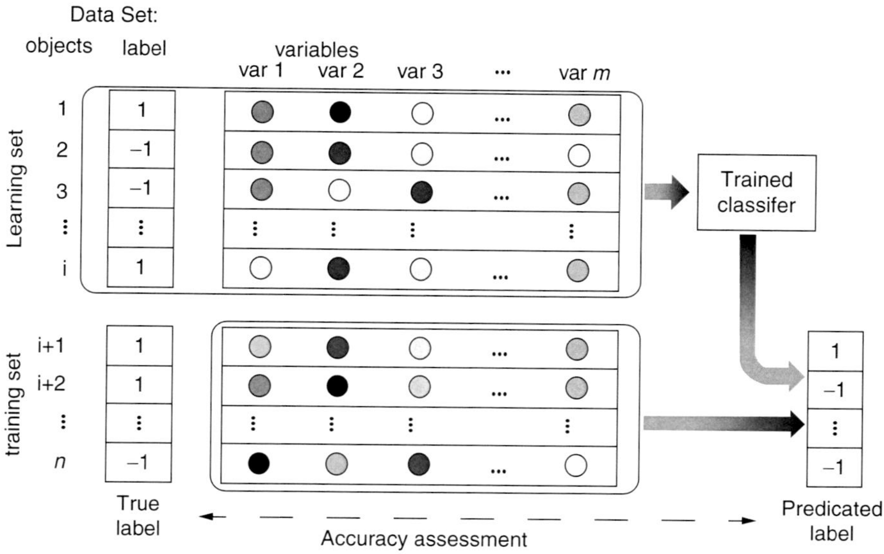

Fig. 4.2 Graphical representation of the data set, split in training and test sets, and of the cross-validation procedure. Each of the n objects or data points is represented by a vector of m variables and its label. The training set, variables and label, is used to train the classifier. The trained classifier is then applied on the test set data and the predicted labels are compared to the true labels to assess the classifier's accuracy

a new input. For the rest of this chapter, we only focus on the discrete classification problem, typically into two categories.

The learning set is generally in the form of a matrix (Fig. 4.2): each "data point" is represented by a vector, which is the collection of variables to feed in the machine, and a label, the output of the function. Usually, the data set comprises n observations or objects to classify, based on the values of m variables. The ratio between the number of objects and the number of variables that describe it plays an important role in the building of the function: if m is large (many variables) compared to n (few observations), then there is a risk of "over-fitting" [14]. If this dimensionality issue, also known as the "curse of dimensionality" [15], is not accounted for properly, the optimized machine can achieve perfect classification on the training data but will classify poorly any new data point: the resulting classifier does not generalize to similar but slightly different data points.

To validate and assess the generalizability of the trained classifier, the data set is usually divided into two parts: the "learning set," on which the classifier is trained, and the "testing set," used to compute the accuracy of the classifier. Depending on the size of the data set available, this training-then-testing procedure can be repeated multiple times with different splits of the data set. The final accuracy of the model is computed as the mean of the model accuracy at each division. This is referred to as "cross-validation procedure."

The accuracy of the model is generally computed in terms of correct or misclassifications for each category (Table 4.1; Eq. 4.1). For example, with the

Table 4.1 Different types of classification errors for the case of two classes

$$\text{Accuracy} = \text{TP} + \text{TN} / (\text{TP} + \text{FP} + \text{FN} + \text{TN}) \quad (4.1)$$

$$\text{Sensitivity} = \text{TP} / (\text{TP} + \text{FN}) \quad (4.2)$$

$$\text{Specificity} = \text{TN} / (\text{TN} + \text{FP}) \quad (4.3)$$

	Class 1 (true label: −1)	Class 2 (true label: +1)
Class 1 (predicted label: −1)	True negative (TN)	False negative (FN)
Class 2 (predicted label: +1)	False positive (FP)	True positive (TP)

The '−1' and '+1' labels correspond to Class 1 and Class 2, respectively, e.g., the absence (−1) or presence (+1) of a disease for a test subject

handwritten digits, 80% classification accuracy for 1's means that four times out of five the trained machine correctly recognizes the handwritten digit, and is incorrect in one case out of five, i.e., the digit "1" is not recognized or another digit is recognized as "1". More specific parameters can also be derived, such as the sensitivity and specificity of the model (Eqs. 4.2 and 4.3), which allows more insight into the characteristics of the classification algorithm. Still, with the handwritten digits to classify, for example, a sensibility of 90% and specificity of 60% would mean that: if "1" is actually handwritten, then it is correctly recognized 9 times out of 10 (1 "false negative") but for any 10 other handwritten digits except "1", 4 of them are erroneously classified as "1" (4 "false positive").

This can be very important, e.g., in the case of pathology classification, it is crucial to correctly detect all diseased patients and limit to a minimum the number of false negatives, i.e., maximize the sensitivity even if it reduces a bit the specificity.

There are many ways of building the input–output function, depending on how the data are mathematically modeled. Among the various existing techniques, common ones are the kernel-based approaches [16] such as support vector machines (SVM) [17], relevant vector machine (RVM) [18], and Gaussian processes (GP) [19] as well as other approaches like linear discriminant analysis [15] or Gaussian naïve bayes [2, 20].

When it comes to applying data mining tools to brain imaging data, SVM is one of the most widespread methods. This technique is based on a simple and logical idea: when discriminating between objects from different categories, the larger the distance between objects from different categories, the better the classification. SVM is mostly a binary classifier, i.e., it discriminates between only two categories of patterns, and thus aims at finding the best hyper-plane separating the data of the two categories, i.e., the margin between data points from each category and the hyper-plane is maximized (as illustrated in Fig. 4.3 for the case of 2D data points). In practice, the data points located on the margin are the only ones defining the hyper-plane and are called "support vectors," hence, the name "support vector machine." SVM (like RVM) is a sparse technique relying on a form of "automatic relevance determination" [21], i.e., the automatic selection of relevant or representative data points among the whole data set.

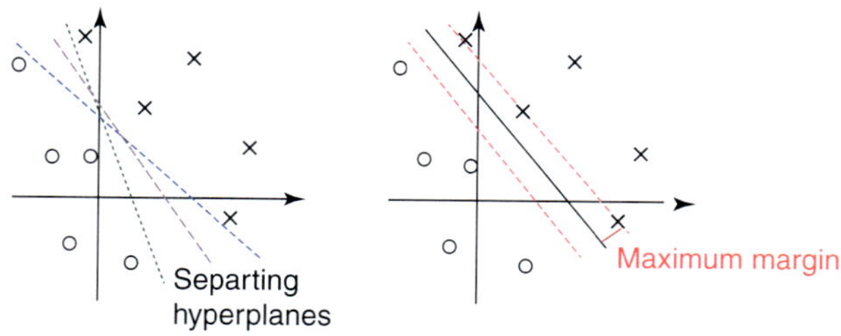

Fig. 4.3 "Support vector machine" principle: The objects considered have two variables, their value being represented by both axes, and come from two categories (× and o here). The object families are separated by a hyper-plane. Among all the possible hyper-planes (three are shown in the *left image*), the one that maximizes the margin (*right image*) is picked up by SVM. The data points on the margin are called "support vectors"

Applications

Data mining tools can be applied to a large variety of data sets, from classification of handwritten digits to classification of brain activity induced by visualized images. The simple form of the required inputs, a vector of variables, leads to this large spectrum of applicability: all objects that can be characterized by a set of variables stacked in a vector can be classified. For example, an fMRI data set consists of a series of 3D images. Each volume can, therefore, be considered as an observation and can be vectorized according to its voxels values. Volumes corresponding to different mental conditions, e.g., watching images of faces versus those of buildings, can then be classified. In a similar way, grey matter density extracted from structural MR images of patients and controls subjects can be classified [22]. Positron emission tomography (PET) images [23] and electro- or magnetoencephalographic (EEG or MEG) data [24] have also been classified using this perspective.

Multivariate decoding of neuroimaging data can be used to achieve two different objectives: firstly and obviously predict the perceptual, cognitive, or medical state of one or many subjects but also, secondly, reveal the pattern of voxels leading to the discrimination of these states. With a linear SVM (and other linear kernel machines), these two goals can be reached simultaneously: the estimated weight associated to each voxel reveals the patterns of voxels considered as important by the model to perform the classification. Or else, the trained machine can be treated as a "black box" that predicts the category of any new data fed in. This last application can be viewed as a diagnostic tool in the case of a disease-versus-healthy classification (or any variation).

Diagnostic Tool

The application of multivariate analysis as a diagnostic tool could become particularly useful, especially, when the concerned disease is difficult to diagnose using classical clinical exams. Alzheimer's disease (AD), one of the commonest causes of dementia, is a good example: a definitive diagnosis of AD can only be obtained using postmortem histopathological analysis. Currently, AD is diagnosed using clinical exams, neuropsychological testing, and manual measurements on brain images (MRI or PET), leading to time-consuming criteria and accuracies of the diagnosis around 80%, at best [25]. AD is, therefore, often misdiagnosed; although an early treatment would be more effective. Multivariate analyses performed on structural MR images of patients and controls allowed the construction of SVM, able to automatically distinguish between healthy subjects and AD patients with accuracies between 86% [22] and 96% [26], depending on the sample size and information used. Moreover, in [26], data from different scanners were used, suggesting that a trained classifier could be applied across centers.

These studies relied on SVM and, therefore, led to binary 0/1 classifications: the input image is classified in one category or the other without further information about the classification reliability. Nevertheless, when using a multivariate technique as a diagnostic tool, knowing the probability associated with the prediction would be very valuable. Consider two new images, from two patients A and B, classified as "healthy," but the one from Patient A has a probability of 99% of being so and the one from B only 51%. In both cases, under a binary classification scheme, the corresponding subjects could be considered as "healthy," but the classification probability of the B image is very close to the "50% chance threshold," which might suggest further exams are needed to confirm or infirm the diagnostic of Patient B.

"Relevance Vector Machine" (RVM), akin to SVM, provides such probabilistic prediction by returning the posterior probability of being in one category versus the other – thanks to its Bayesian formulation. RVM was recently applied on fluorodeoxyglucose PET (FDG-PET) data, i.e., images of cerebral glucose metabolism of patients (vegetative state: VS, and locked-in syndrome: LIS) and healthy controls [23].

First, an RVM was trained to discriminate VS patients ($n=13$) from healthy subjects ($n=37$) using their FDG-PET images. With these well-defined and separate categories, i.e., unconscious versus conscious subjects, cross-validation of this "consciousness classifier" showed 100% accuracy. Then, the trained RVM was applied on the FDG-PET images of eight LIS patients: the probabilities returned ranged between 61% and 100% to be in the "conscious" category. This suggests that LIS patients could be automatically and correctly classified as conscious, contrary to VS patients, based only on the patterns of their cerebral metabolism.

Relevant Patterns of Voxels

In the case of a linear kernel classifier, the relevance of each voxel can be estimated as a weighted linear combination of the same voxel values of the images used for training. This "voxel relevance" is not a statistical value, per se, but simply reflects how much any voxel contributes to the classification of the input image into one output category or the other: a large (respectively small) value (in absolute value)

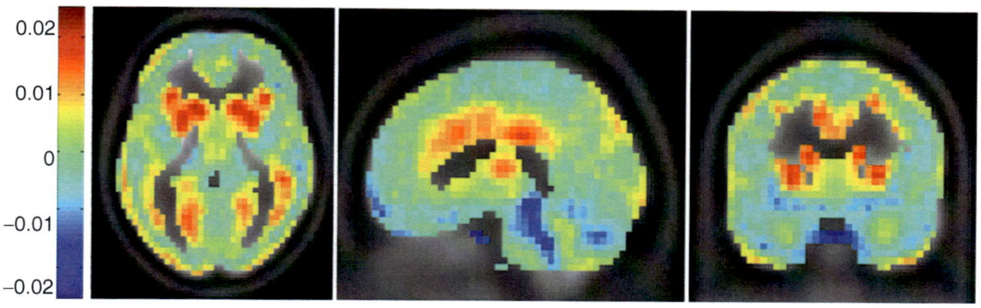

Fig. 4.4 Distribution over the brain volume of the voxel relevance for a " relevance vector machine" trained to discriminate between FDG-PET images of VS patients and healthy subjects. A positive value (*yellow–red*) indicates that relatively large metabolic activity in those voxels will drive the classification towards the "healthy subject" category. Conversely, negative values (*blue–purple*) pushes towards the "VS patient" category. The voxels with little relevance (*green*) hardly contribute to the classification of data (Adapted from Phillips et al. [23])

indicates that this voxel has relatively much (respectively little) influence on the classification. Since there is a value per voxel, it is possible to present a "relevance map" as an image in brain space (see Fig. 4.4 for the relevance maps of the control versus VS classification) [23]. Such a map can bring insight on the location of the discriminating areas and, therefore, help neuroscientists build more efficient criteria of diagnosis but also orient them during the elaboration of new hypotheses concerning the origins or evolution of a certain disease or disorder.

Perspectives

In view of the recent advances in multivariate pattern analysis, these techniques certainly will become more common to study consciousness. Their application as a diagnostic tool to differentiate patients presents obvious advantages such as objectiveness, automation, and the fact that a posterior probability can be provided with the final prediction, compared to current time-consuming and subjective criteria.

Other applications could also be envisaged, e.g., classification techniques could be applied to "response to command" experiences in fMRI [27], leading to reproducible user-independent and possibly more accurate results than the current "general linear model" analysis used. Furthermore, multivariate analysis could be applied online as the data are acquired, i.e., during the recording – the model is updated in real-time with each new image. Online processing of "response to command" fMRI experiments offers a new communication channel relying solely on brain activation [28]. Such "brain–computer interface" schemes could certainly benefit, in term of accuracy and speed, from more advanced "brain decoding" tools.

Finally, "brain reading" could, maybe one day, offer a partial view on the mental content of patients in altered states of consciousness. First, a model would be trained with data acquired from healthy subjects thinking about different semantic categories of pictures and words, e.g., faces, buildings, animals or emotions [29]. Then, this model would be applied on data from minimally conscious state or VS patients.

References

1. Ogawa S, Lee TM, Kay AR, Tank DW. Brain magnetic resonance imaging with contrast dependent on bloodoxygenation. Proc Nat Acad Sci USA. 1990;87:9868–72.
2. Friston KJ, Ashburner JT, Kiebel SJ, et al. Statistical parametric mapping: the analysis of functional brain images. London/Burlington, San Diego: Elsevier/Academic Press; 2007.
3. Holmes A, Poline JB, Friston KJ. Characterizing brain images with the general linear model. In: Human brain function. San Diego: Academic Press; 1997. p. 59–84.
4. Norman KA, Polyn SM, Detre GJ, Haxby JV. Beyond mind-reading: multi-voxel pattern analysis of fMRI data. Trends Cogn Sci. 2008;10:424–30.
5. Friston K, Chu C, Mourão-Miranda J, et al. Bayesian decoding of brain images. Neuroimage. 2008;39:181–205.
6. Haynes JD, Rees G. Decoding mental states from brain activity in humans. Nat Rev Neurosci. 2006;7:523–34.
7. Spiridon M, Kanwisher N. How distributed is visual category information in human occipito-temporal cortex? An fMRI study. Neuron. 2002;35:1157–65.
8. Cox DD, Savoy RL. Functional magnetic resonance imaging (fMRI) 'brain reading': detecting and classifying distributed patterns of fMRI activity in human visual cortex. Neuroimage. 2003;19:261–70.
9. Shinkareva S, Mason RA, Malave VL, et al. Using fMRI brain activation to identify cognitive states associated with perception of tools and dwellings. PLoS One. 2008;3(3):1394.
10. Kamitani Y, Tong F. Decoding the visual and subjective contents of the human brain. Nat Neurosci. 2005;8:679–85.
11. Haynes J, Rees G. Predicting the orientation of invisible stimuli from activity in human primary visual cortex. Nat Neurosci. 2005;8:686–91.
12. Polyn S, Natu V, Cohen J, Norman K. Category-specific cortical activity precedes retrieval during memory search. Science. 2005;310:1963–6.
13. Chadwick M, Hassabis D, Weiskopf N, Maguire E. Decoding individual episodic memory traces in the human hippocampus. Curr Biol. 2010;20:1–4.
14. Pitt MA, Myung IJ. When a good fit can be bad. Trends Cogn Sci. 2002;6:421–5.
15. Bishop CM. Pattern recognition and machine learning. Springer; 2006. http://www.springer.com/computer/image+processing/book/978-0-387-31073-2
16. Müller KR, Mika S, Rätsch G, et al. An introduction to kernel-based learning algorithms. IEEE Trans Neural Netw. 2001;12:181–202.
17. Burges C. A tutorial on support vector machines for pattern recognition. Data Mining Knowl Discov. 1998;2:121–67.
18. Tipping ME. Sparse Bayesian learning and the relevance vector machine. J Mach Learn Res. 2001;1:211–44.
19. Rasmussen CE, Williams CKI. Gaussian processes for machine learning. Cambridge: The MIT Press; 2006.
20. Mitchell TM, Hutchinson R, Niculescu RS, et al. Learning to decode cognitive states from brain images. Mach Learn. 2004;57:145–75.
21. Neal RM. Bayesian learning for neural networks. New York: Springer; 1996.
22. Vemuri P, Gunter JL, Senjem ML, et al. Alzheimer's disease diagnosis in individual subjects using structural MR images: validation studies. Neuroimage. 2008;39:1186–97.

23. Phillips C, Bruno MA, Maquet P, et al. "Relevance vector machine" consciousness classifier applied to cerebral metabolism of vegetative and locked-in patients. Neuroimage. 15 May 2011;56(2):797–808.
24. Chan AM, Halgren E, Marinkovic K, Cash SS. Decoding word and category-specific spatiotemporal representations from MEG and EEG. Neuroimage. 2011;54:3028–39.
25. Knopman DS, DeKosky ST, Cummings JL, et al. Practice parameter: diagnosis of dementia (an evidence-based review). report of the quality standards Subcommittee of the American Academy of Neurology. Neurology. 2001;56:1143–53.
26. Kloppel S, Stonnington CM, Chu C, et al. Automatic classification of MR scans in Alzheimer's disease. Brain. 2008;131:681–9.
27. Monti MM, Vanhaudenhuyse A, Coleman MR, et al. Willful modulation of brain activity in disorders of consciousness. N Engl J Med. 2010;362:579–89.
28. Sorger B, Dahmen B, Reithler J, et al. Another kind of 'BOLD response': answering multiple-choice questions via online decoded single-trial brain signals. In: Progress in brain research. Vol 177. Elsevier; 2009. p. 275–92. http://www.elsevier.com/wps/find/bookdescription.cws_home/720425/description#description
29. Mitchell TM, Shinkareva SV, Carlson A, et al. Predicting human brain activity associated with the meanings of nouns. Science. 2008;30:1191–5.

Chapter 5
Spectroscopy and Diffusion Tensor Imaging in Disorders of Consciousness

Jean-Flory Luaba Tshibanda, Athena Demertzi, and Andrea Soddu

Introduction

Medical advances in (neuro) intensive care currently allow patients suffering from severe brain lesions, such as traumatic brain injury or anoxia, to survive. These patients can evolve toward brain death, a vegetative state, a minimally conscious state, or toward recovery of normal consciousness level [1]. In most cases, this evolution is based on behavioral testing, which is explained in Chapter 1. This examination implies a part of subjectivity and does not always lead to an accurate diagnosis. It has been shown that about 40% of patients considered as being in a vegetative state were, in fact, in a minimally conscious state when assessed more carefully [2–4]. This high rate of misdiagnosis is unacceptable for all medical and paramedical professionals in-charge and (might influence) for the efficacy of the patient's management, the accuracy of the information provided to the family, and the balanced management of financial resources. On the other hand, a consensus on end-of-life decisions has to be considered as regards the debates currently happening within the medical field.

Magnetic resonance imaging (MRI) may help to improve the diagnosis of patients with disorders of consciousness and provide prognosis of the recovery of patients' brain functioning. This technique allows not only a better assessment of structural lesions but also a better understanding of disorders of consciousness.

J.-F.L. Tshibanda, M.D. (✉)
Coma Science Group, Cyclotron Research Center, University of Liège,
Allée du 6 Août, Sart Tilman B30, 4000 Liège, Belgium

Department of Radiology, University Hospital of Liège,
Liège, Belgium
e-mail: l.tshibanda@chu.ulg.ac.be

A. Demertzi, M.Sc. • A. Soddu, Ph.D.
Coma Science Group, Cyclotron Research Center, University of Liège,
Allée du 6 Août, Sart Tilman B30, 4000 Liège, Belgium

C. Schnakers, S. Laureys (eds.), *Coma and Disorders of Consciousness*,
DOI 10.1007/978-1-4471-2440-5_5, © Springer-Verlag London 2012

Magnetic Resonance Imaging

Technological advances of these last 10 years in the field of magnetic resonance imaging have radically changed our understanding of coma and of post-comatose states of consciousness.

MRI techniques allow the realization of structural, metabolic, and functional measures of brain structures involved in arousal and awareness. These refer to the reticular activating system located in the posterior upper part of the pons, the cerebral peduncles, the thalamus, the hypothalamus, the inferior part of the frontal lobes, and the precuneus [5–9]. A good knowledge of brain lesions caused by traumatic brain injury and stroke, which are the main etiologies responsible for impairments of consciousness, will allow clinicians to choose adequately the MRI sequences. Traumatic brain injury causes brain contusions and diffuse axonal lesions. Contusions (often located in temporal and frontal areas) are the consequence of the impact of the parenchyma against the skull; while diffuse axonal lesions are caused by rotational acceleration–deceleration events. These axonal lesions are often located between structures of different density, such as the juxtacortical or periventricular white matter, the corpus callosum, the basal ganglia, and the brainstem (midbrain and pons). These lesions can be ischemic or hemorrhagic, which can influence the prognosis of posttraumatic cerebral functioning. Anoxic/hypoxic lesions resulting from a stroke are often accompanied by a cytotoxic edema. These lesions can evolve toward recovery or toward tissue necrosis and hemorrhage.

It is important to choose the right moment to scan a patient recovering from coma in order to benefit from an MRI examination. An MRI scan performed in a strict dorsal decubitus can lead to intracranial hypertension in acute patients suffering a severe brain injury. Additionally, this technique can allow the detection of reversible lesions such as edema; but can miss secondary brain lesions (linked to the patient's global deterioration or linked to the presence of intracranial hypertension), which are likely to aggravate the functional prognosis of the brain [10–12]. On the other hand, a late MRI examination allows the detection of sequels and atrophies [13]; but has no impact on the patient's treatment or on the prognostic value. The ideal moment for a MRI scan seems to be the third week after the brain edema disappears [14].

A three-dimensional T1 sequence is performed in order to estimate cerebral atrophy and is used as an anatomical reference for the areas of cortical activation observed with functional imaging. The "fluid attenuated inversion recovery" (FLAIR) sequence is useful to detect ischemic lesions, contusions, and diffuse axonal (not hemorrhagic) lesions. These lesions are often invisible using tomodensitometry and can explain disorders of consciousness in those patients where tomodensitometrical results were normal. Diffuse axonal hemorrhagic lesions are revealed by the T2* sequence, which shows microbleedings as well as hypointense lesions, due to the presence of hemosiderin (Fig. 5.1). The number of lesions detected by these two morphological T2* sequences is correlated to patients' long-term prognosis [15, 16]. The prognosis is particularly negative in the case of bilateral lesions involving the brainstem [17, 18]. Although these two sequences are very sensitive in the detection of lesions, they do not explain disorders of consciousness presented by patients who do not show any

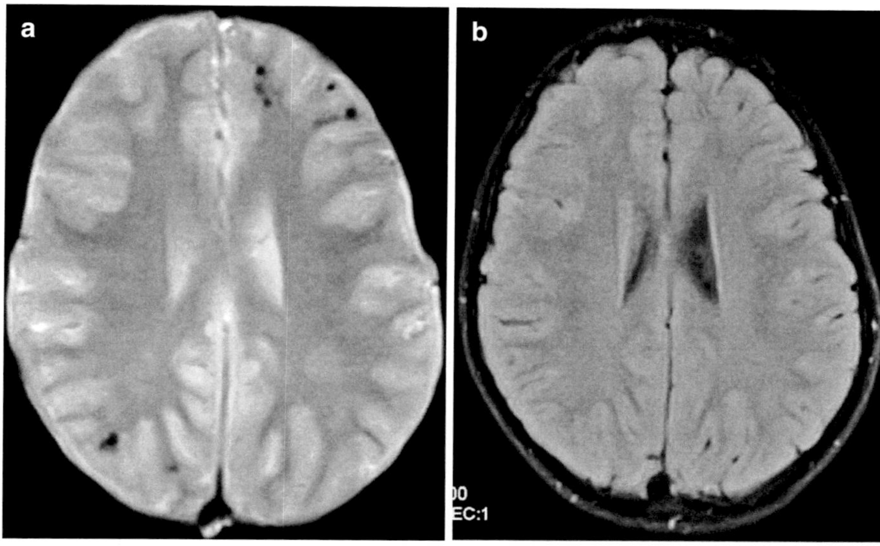

Fig. 5.1 Traumatic patient in a minimally conscious state. The axial T2* sequence images (**a**) show hemorrhagic diffuse axonal lesions invisible on the axial FLAIR sequence images (**b**)

abnormality of the brainstem. Therefore, they are not sufficient to establish a prognosis. There is, hence, a growing interest for using innovative techniques, such as spectroscopy, tensor imaging, or functional imaging.

Magnetic Resonance Spectroscopy

In contrast to conventional MRI, which provides anatomical information based on the tissue water signal, magnetic resonance spectroscopy (MRS) provides chemical information based on the signal of tissue metabolites. Atoms studied in vivo with MRS are proton (1H), phosphorus (31P), carbon (13C), sodium (23NA), potassium (39K), and fluorine (19F).

Spectroscopy of proton conduction is currently the most used technique in the exploration of post-comatose disorders of consciousness. Conducted with a 1.5 or 3 T MRI, this noninvasive technique allows the study of the brain function by the quantification of several metabolites. The detection of these metabolites constitutes a real challenge, considering their very weak concentration in comparison to peri- and intracerebral water. This problem is solved by using techniques that allow the abolition of the tissue water signal. Besides, the heterogeneity of the parenchyma thickness requires focal measurements, which lead to use voxels of 1 or 2 cm^3 and to a low signal-to-noise ratio. The MRS performed in vivo with abolition of the tissue water signal and with a 135 or 270 ms echo-time focuses on four metabolites: [1] Choline (Cho), appearing at 3.2 ppm, is a marker of membrane synthesis and catabolism and is more abundant in white matter than in gray matter. Its rate increases in case of cell proliferation, in inflammatory and demyelinating processes; [2] Creatine (Cr), appearing at 3.0 ppm, is a relatively stable marker of aerobic energetic metabolism; [3] The *N*-acetyl-aspartate (NAA), appearing at 2.0 ppm, is present in neural cytoplasm and in axons. The NAA is equally distributed in gray and white matter [19]. Several studies suggest that this metabolite is a cerebral osmolytes likely to introduce reversible variations [20, 21]. It is reduced in all diseases that are accompanied by neural or axonal loss, such as neurodegenerative pathologies, stroke, traumatic brain injury, and glial tumors; and, hence, is a marker of neural and axonal integrity [22]. The possibility to quantify neural damages in vivo is certainly one of the most important applications of the MRS; and [4] lactate, appearing at 1.3 ppm, is a marker of anaerobic metabolism and is usually difficult to detect. Its rate increases in case of hypoxia, ischemia, or severe traumatic injury.

The exploration of post-comatose patients includes two MRS acquisitions. A sequence of mono-voxel proton MRS (single voxel spectroscopy or SVS) is performed at the level of the posterior upper section of the pons (Fig. 5.2) as it contains the reticular activating system known for its role in arousal. Besides, the pons is often damaged by diffuse axonal lesions invisible on FLAIR and T2* sequences and can detect secondary lesions due to a temporal herniation. A multi-voxel proton MRS (chemical shift imaging or CSI) is performed at the level of the basal ganglia and allows assessing metabolites in several anatomical structures involved in arousal and awareness processes, such as thalami, lenticular nucleus, mesiofrontal areas, and occipital periventricular white matter (Fig. 5.3). The difficulty in conducting an absolute quantification of these metabolites leads to use values based on the ratio of a metabolite divided by the sum of metabolites or by another metabolite considered to be stable. Creatine plays the role of reference to calculate the NAA/Cr or Cho/Cr ratios. A recent review has underlined several studies showing the efficacy of the MRS in predicting recovery of brain-injured patients [23], confirming the preliminary study of Choe et al. [24], who suggested that the decrease of NAA/Cr ratio could underline axonal loss in the case of traumatic brain injury and could constitute a metabolic criterion for recovery in these patients. Usually, NAA/Cr ratio is superior or equal to 1.50 and NAA/NAA + Cho + Cr ratio is equal to 0.40.

In case of traumatic brain injury, a reduction of the NAA/Cr ratio is a reliable indicator of negative prognosis [25]. This ratio decreases rapidly few hours after the onset and reaches its lowest value within 48 h. It remains stable for a month afterward allowing the realization of MRI scans in the third week postinjury when the cerebral edema has decreased. It, nevertheless, strongly fluctuates 6 weeks to 1 year postinjury. Within this period of time, some authors observed a constant reduction of NAA/Cr ratio [26, 27] while others observed a biphasic evolution (i.e., increase/decrease phase) of this one [28]. The variability of the NAA/Cr ratio is a potential limit of this technology. Moreover, the use of creatine as a reliable reference to calculate the values of NAA and Cho stresses the problem of stability of creatine concentration. Indeed, it is not established that creatine remains stable in the case of traumatic brain injury. Some studies showed that its concentration can increase in hypometabolic states and decrease in hypermetabolic states [29, 30].

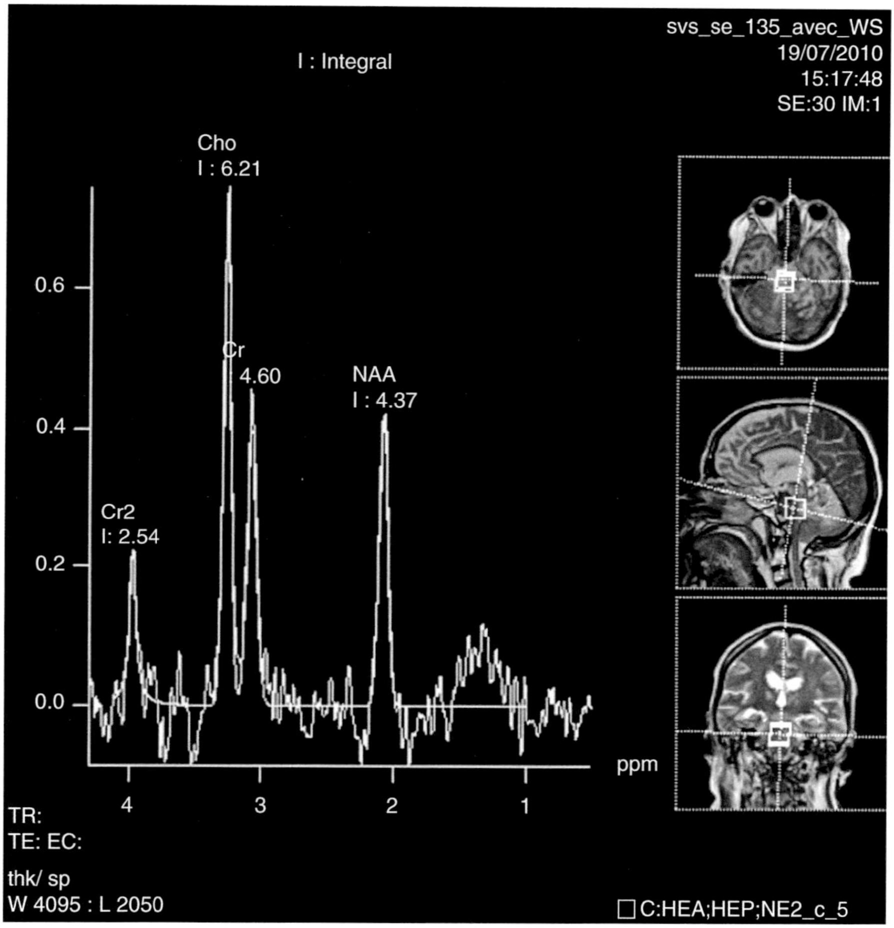

Fig. 5.2 Vegetative patient. The sequence of single voxel spectroscopy (*SVS*) performed in the pons shows a decrease of the NAA/Cr ratio

The MRS contributes to improve the establishment of functional prognosis of severe brain-injured patients and permits to follow their clinical evolution in parallel to the NAA/Cr ratio, a decrease of this ratio being indicative of poor prognosis.

Diffusion Tensor Imaging

Diffusion tensor imaging (DTI) is an MRI technique that allows the study in vivo of tissue microstructure, which was developed based on the study of the diffusion of water molecules. This diffusion is free when molecules randomly move in a

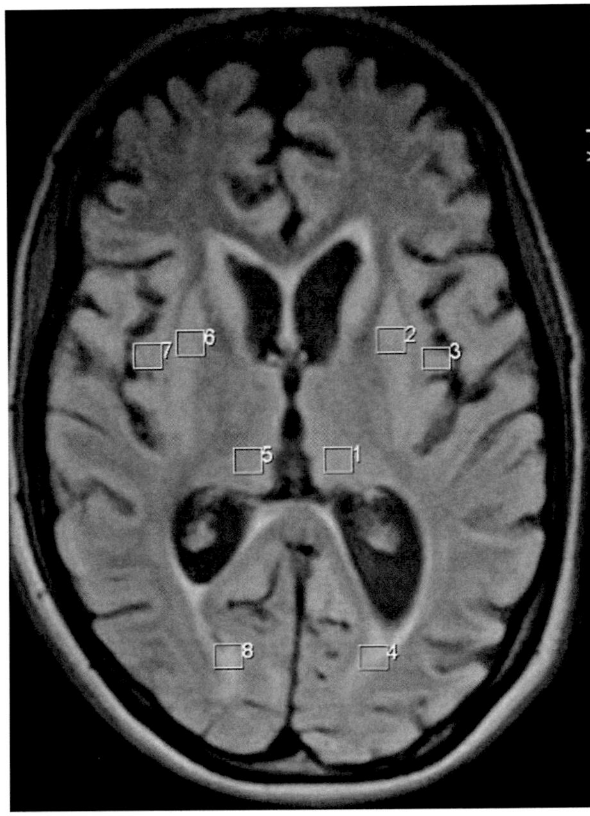

Fig. 5.3 Illustration of the areas where the metabolites are measured using chemical shift imaging (*CSI*): thalamus, lenticular nucleus, insula and periventricular white matter

homogeneous environment without restriction such as the cerebrospinal fluid (Brownian motion). Restricted isotropic diffusion happens when the movement of water molecules is restricted in all directions and restricted anisotropic diffusion happens when this restriction is only present in some directions, creating heterogeneity in the speed of movements of water molecules or anisotropy. The axonal organization is at the origin of anisotropic diffusion in the white matter – the diffusion of water molecules is preferentially directed in parallel to the axon and restricted perpendicularly to this one. The detection of water diffusion direction around axons allows the study of functional connectivity. It is, hence, possible to study cognitive deficits according to the anatomical connectivity between brain areas coding for these cognitive processes.

Diffusion tensor imaging allows measuring the fractional anisotropy (FA). Its value is equal to zero when the diffusion is isotropic or is high when the diffusion is anisotropic. It allows creating a map of the white matter with color codification for the orientation of axons (Fig. 5.4). The diffusion tensor imaging is the only technique giving in vivo overview of the axonal tracts (tractography). In case of disorders of consciousness, the FA is measured in the posterior section of the pons, in the cerebral peduncles, in the internal and external capsules, in the periventricular white matter, and in the semioval center (Fig. 5.4). The destruction of the axons leads to a reduction of the anisotropic diffusion and, therefore, of the FA. This one constitutes a noninvasive marker of the integrity of axonal tracts using T2* and FLAIR sequences [31]. The study performed by Perlbarg et al. [32] showed a reduction of the FA measured in the cerebral peduncles, the internal capsule, and the corpus callosum in the group of traumatic brain injured patients with a bad outcome as compared to those with a good outcome. By studying the recovery of traumatic patients at 1 year postonset, Tollard et al. [33] observed a reduction of FA in all measured brain areas. They also noticed that combining spectroscopy (NAA, Cr) and diffusion (FA) methods allowed the prediction of bad outcome at 1 year with a specificity of 97% against 75% only for the spectroscopy and 85% only for the diffusion. For the three cases, the sensitivity is, respectively, 86%, 75%, and 79%. These two studies confirm that the FA constitutes a good biomarker for detecting lesions in the white matter.

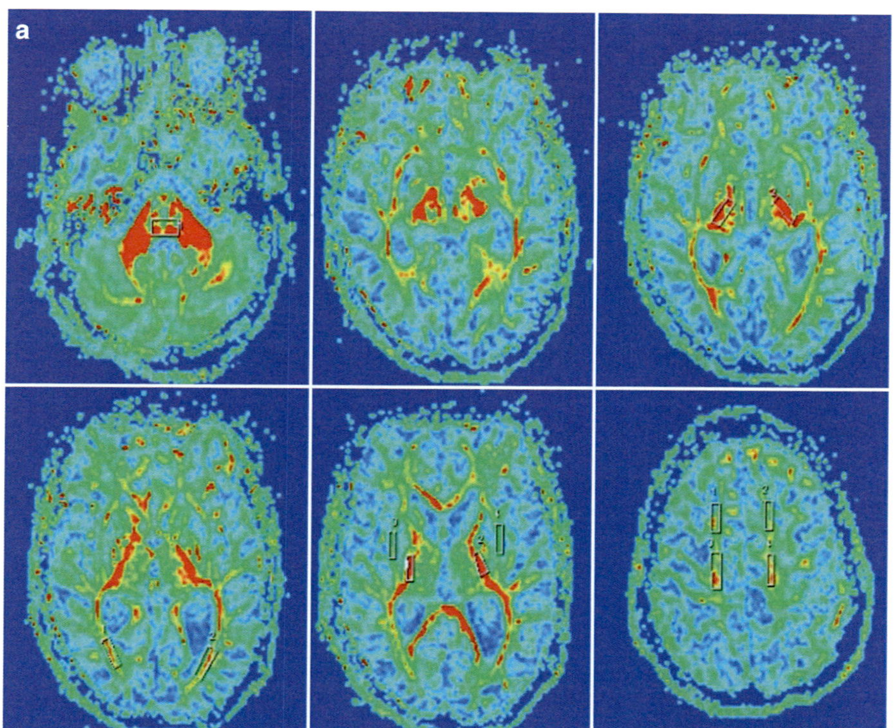

Fig. 5.4 (**a**) Diffusion tensor imaging with color codification for the axonal orientation. (**b**) Illustration of the areas where the fractional anisotropy (*FA*) is measured: pons, cerebral peduncles, internal and external capsules, periventricular white matter and semioval center

Fig. 5.4 (continued)

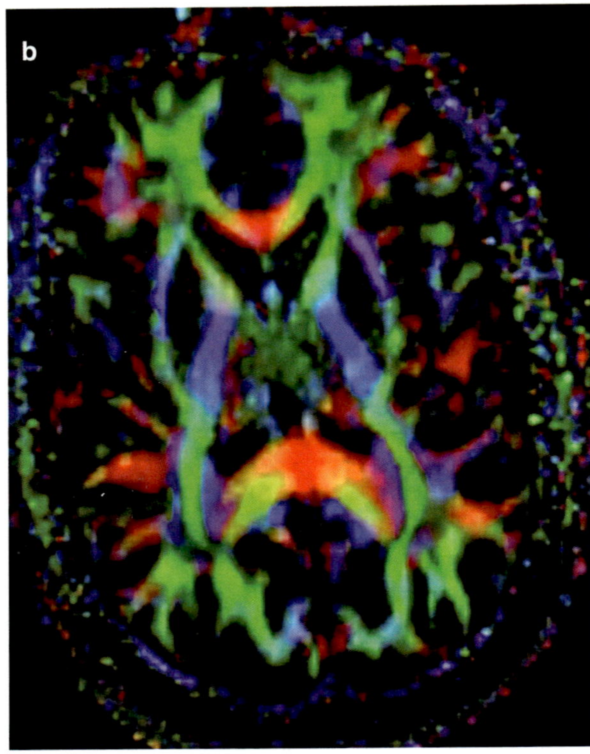

Conclusions

Spectroscopy and diffusion tensor imaging detect invisible tissue lesions using FLAIR and T2* sequences. These techniques allow a better diagnosis and prognosis of patients with disorders of consciousness (particularly, when they are combined) and permit a better monitoring of the deterioration or recovery of posttraumatic brain functioning by considering the fluctuation of the NAA/Cr and FA values in time. To our mind, in the future, these noninvasive techniques will play a more important role in the monitoring of post-comatose patients.

References

1. Laureys S, Boly M. The changing spectrum of coma. Nat Clin Pract Neurol. 2008;4:544–6.
2. Childs NL, Mercer WN, Childs HW. Accuracy of diagnosis of persistent vegetative state. Neurology. 1993;43:1465–7.
3. Andrews K, Murphy L, Munday R, et al. Misdiagnosis of the vegetative state: retrospective study in a rehabilitation unit. BMJ. 1996;313:13–6.
4. Schnakers C, Vanhaudenhuyse A, Giacino J, et al. Diagnostic accuracy of the vegetative and minimally conscious state: clinical consensus versus standardized neurobehavioral assessment. BMC Neurol. 2009;9:35.

5. Kampfl A, Schmutzhard E, Franz G, et al. Prediction of recovery from post-traumatic vegetative state with cerebral magnetic-resonance imaging. Lancet. 1998;351:1763–7.
6. Shibata Y, Matsumura A, Meguro K, et al. Differentiation of mechanism and prognosis of traumatic brain stem lesions detected by magnetic resonance imaging in the acute stage. Clin Neurol Neurosurg. 2000;102:124–8.
7. Firsching R, Woischneck D, Klein S, et al. Brain stem lesions after head injury. Neurol Res. 2002;24:145–6.
8. Uzan M, Albayram S, Dashti SG, et al. Thalamic proton magnetic resonance spectroscopy in vegetative state induced by traumatic brain injury. J Neurol Neurosurg Psychiatry. 2003;74:33–8.
9. Salazar AM, Grafman JH, Vance SC, et al. Consciousness and amnesia after penetrating head injury: neurology and anatomy. Neurology. 1986;36:178–87.
10. Huisman TA, Schwamm LH, Schaefer PW, et al. Diffusion tensor imaging as potential biomarker of white matter injury in diffuse axonal injury. AJNR Am J Neuroradiol. 2004;25:370–6.
11. Ross BD, Ernst T, Kreis R, et al. 1H MRS in acute traumatic brain injury. J Magn Reson Imaging. 1998;8:829–40.
12. Marino S, Zei E, Battaglini M, et al. Acute metabolic brain changes following traumatic brain injury and their relevance to clinical severity and outcome. J Neurol Neurosurg Psychiatry. 2007;78:501–7.
13. Trivedi MA, Ward MA, Hess TM, et al. Longitudinal changes in global brain volume between 79 and 409 days after traumatic brain injury: relationship with duration of coma. J Neurotrauma. 2007;24:766–71.
14. Weiss N, Galanaud D, Carpentier A, et al. Clinical review: prognostic value of magnetic resonance imaging in acute brain injury and coma. Crit Care. 2007;11:230.
15. Carpentier A, Galanaud D, Puybasset L, et al. Early morphologic and spectroscopic magnetic resonance in severe traumatic brain injuries can detect "invisible brain stem damage" and predict "vegetative states". J Neurotrauma. 2006;23:674–85.
16. Yanagawa Y, Tsushima Y, Tokumaru A, et al. A quantitative analysis of head injury using T2*-weighted gradient-echo imaging. J Trauma. 2000;49:272–7.
17. Wedekind C, Fischbach R, Pakos P, et al. Comparative use of magnetic resonance imaging and electrophysiologic investigation for the prognosis of head injury. J Trauma. 1999;47:44–9.
18. Firsching R, Woischneck D, Diedrich M, et al. Early magnetic resonance imaging of brainstem lesions after severe head injury. J Neurosurg. 1998;89:707–12.
19. Danielsen ER, Ross B. Magnetic resonance spectroscopy diagnosis of neurological diseases. 1st ed. New York: Marcel Dekker, Inc; 1999.
20. Baslow MH, Suckow RF, Gaynor K, et al. Brain damage results in down-regulation of N-acetylaspartate as a neuronal osmolyte. Neuromolecular Med. 2003;3:95–104.
21. Moffett JR, Ross B, Arun P, et al. N-acetylaspartate in the CNS: from neurodiagnostics to neurobiology. Prog Neurobiol. 2007;81:89–131.
22. Sullivan EV, Adalsteinsson E, Spielman DM, et al. N-acetylaspartate–a marker of neuronal integrity. Ann Neurol. 2001;50:823. author reply 4–5.
23. Tshibanda L, Vanhaudenhuyse A, Galanaud D, et al. Magnetic resonance spectroscopy and diffusion tensor imaging in coma survivors: promises and pitfalls. Prog Brain Res. 2009;177:215–29.
24. Choe BY, Suh TS, Choi KH, et al. Neuronal dysfunction in patients with closed head injury evaluated by in vivo 1 H magnetic resonance spectroscopy. Invest Radiol. 1995;30:502–6.
25. Cecil KM, Hills EC, Sandel ME, et al. Proton magnetic resonance spectroscopy for detection of axonal injury in the splenium of the corpus callosum of brain-injured patients. J Neurosurg. 1998;88:795–801.
26. Garnett MR, Blamire AM, Corkill RG, et al. Early proton magnetic resonance spectroscopy in normal-appearing brain correlates with outcome in patients following traumatic brain injury. Brain. 2000;123(Pt 10):2046–54.
27. Holshouser BA, Tong KA, Ashwal S, et al. Prospective longitudinal proton magnetic resonance spectroscopic imaging in adult traumatic brain injury. J Magn Reson Imaging. 2006;24:33–40.

28. Brooks WM, Stidley CA, Petropoulos H, et al. Metabolic and cognitive response to human traumatic brain injury: a quantitative proton magnetic resonance study. J Neurotrauma. 2000;17:629–40.
29. Castillo M, Kwock L, Mukherji SK. Clinical applications of proton MR spectroscopy. AJNR Am J Neuroradiol. 1996;17:1–15.
30. Wood SJ, Berger G, Velakoulis D, et al. Proton magnetic resonance spectroscopy in first episode psychosis and ultra high-risk individuals. Schizophr Bull. 2003;29:831–43.
31. Huisman T, Sorensen A, Hergan K, et al. Diffusion-weighted imaging for the evaluation of diffuse axonal injury in closed head injury. J Comput Assist Tomogr. 2003;27:5–11.
32. Perlbarg V, Puybasset L, Tollard E, et al. Relation between brain lesion location and clinical outcome in patients with severe traumatic brain injury: a diffusion tensor imaging study using voxel-based approaches. Hum Brain Mapp. 2009;30:3924–33.
33. Tollard E, Galanaud D, Perlbarg V, et al. Experience of diffusion tensor imaging and 1H spectroscopy for outcome prediction in severe traumatic brain injury: preliminary results. Crit Care Med. 2009;37:1448–55.

Chapter 6
Electrophysiology and Disorders of Consciousness

Quentin Noirhomme and Rémy Lehembre

Electroencephalography

Electroencephalography is the measure of the brain's electrical activity using electrodes placed on the surface of the skull. It directly reflects neuronal activity with a high temporal resolution. However, the spatial resolution is poor for two main reasons: (1) it is limited by interelectrode distance and (2) because of volume conduction, each sensor measures a sum of different brain sources, hence sensors have a correlated signal. The number of electrodes used depends on the application. For instance, when monitoring the level of anesthesia, only two electrodes are needed to obtain an electroencephalographic trace, while in clinical environments at least ten are used. In research, modern electrode caps have up to 256 electrodes. Electrode positioning on the cranial surface follows international nomenclatures (10–20 system for up to 19 electrodes and 10–10 system for more than 19 electrodes [1]), which aim to cover homogeneously most of the cranial surface. Electrodes are named according to their position on the scalp and have the letter F for frontal, C for central, P for parietal, O for occipital, or a letter combination such as FC for a position between frontal and central. Additionally, these letters are followed by a number (even for electrodes on the right hemisphere and odd for electrodes on the left hemisphere) or by the letter Z (for electrodes on the midline).

The measured signal results from a potential difference between two electrodes. It is, therefore, not possible to use only one electrode. There are two categories of montages: bipolar montages in which the electrodes are paired two by two; and

Q. Noirhomme, Ph.D. (✉) • R. Lehembre, M.Sc.
Coma Science Group, Cyclotron Research Centre, University of Liège,
Allée du 6 Août 8, Sart Tilman B30, 4000 Liège, Belgium
e-mail: quentin.noirhomme@ulg.ac.be; remy.lehembre@ulg.ac.be

C. Schnakers, S. Laureys (eds.), *Coma and Disorders of Consciousness*,
DOI 10.1007/978-1-4471-2440-5_6, © Springer-Verlag London 2012

referential montages where all the electrodes are coupled to a single electrode called the reference. In a bipolar montage, it can be considered that the recorded signal stems from an imaginary position located between the two electrodes. In a referential montage, the reference should not be located in a region where a signal of interest has to be recorded. Common positions for the reference are the ear lobes, the mastoids, possibly coupled, the nose, or a position on the midline. The choice of the reference electrode has an influence on the shape of the recorded signal, notably for evoked potentials. Bipolar montages are less sensitive to artifacts but will not detect events that are common to two coupled electrodes. A referential montage does not have this drawback but is, however, more sensitive to artifacts [2].

The electroencephalogram (EEG) does not only detect electrical fields generated by cerebral activity but also fields generated by muscular activity such as eye or eyelids movements, or fields generated by electrical apparatus. Patients in altered states of consciousness are often surrounded by many different electronic equipments withstanding their vital functions. They have little control of their movements and can be spastic. Furthermore, they do not control their level of sudation, which can potentially be the cause of artifacts, which should be minimized during the recording. It is good practice to simultaneously record respiration, heartbeats, and muscular activity in order to better track artifacts and eventually remove them from the signal. It is also important to have full knowledge of all drugs prescribed to the patient as some can have a sedative effect, which can result in a slower EEG, or others such as benzodiazepines can add additional fast frequencies to the signal. Some artifacts can be eliminated by data filtering. A notch filter removes the 50 Hz line noise (60 Hz in the United States and other regions in the world). The EEG spectrum covers frequencies ranging from less than 1 Hz to several hundreds of Hz. The use of filters should, therefore, depend on the frequency bands of interest. Too much filtering of low frequencies might hide slow waves activity while filtering high frequencies might hide spindles and spike waves. Heavy filtering results in a clean EEG trace but might remove some of the signal of interest [2]. Taking these considerations into account, the EEG signal is often observed after filtering between 1 and 30 Hz, notably in sleep studies or for evoked potentials. These limits can then be adjusted in order to include more frequencies.

There are three main approaches in the study of EEG, which are presented in separate sections. The first approach consists in the visual inspection of the electroencephalographic trace in order to unveil background EEG activity and characteristic events. It gives global information on cerebral activity. The second approach, based on evoked potentials, measures the brain's response to an external stimulation such as a sound or a flash. It is useful in the study of auditory, visual, or sensory–motor areas. Finally, the third approach is quantitative and aims to extract characteristic EEG features of cerebral activity. Such features are, e.g., the power in different frequency bands, an index of wakefulness, or a measure of connectivity between cerebral areas. The goal of this approach is to provide an automated EEG analysis, but it is still under development.

EEG Interpretation

The visual interpretation of an EEG trace gives information on the global cerebral activity of a patient. The EEG can help to establish the origin and the severity of the injury (e.g., in the case of a focal lesion or a diffuse dysfunction) and differentiate states that are apparently similar to coma such as an epileptic absence, a psychogenic coma, a noncooperative patient, or a locked-in syndrome. Combined with the etiology, the EEG can give an indication on the patient's prognosis. Finally, the EEG can track the patient evolution and the effect of drugs such as anti-epileptics [3–5].

The EEG of a control subject is mainly composed of an alpha rhythm (8–12 Hz) with a posterior and symmetric distribution. Its amplitude increases when the subject is resting and eyes closed. An additional beta rhythm (13–30 Hz) of smaller amplitude can be irregularly observed. These rhythms are underlined by slower rhythms which are more visible when the subject becomes tired. In tired subjects, a theta rhythm (4–7 Hz) becomes the dominant rhythm. Once asleep, subjects have a predominance of delta rhythms (1–3 Hz). In patients with disorders of consciousness, a slower EEG can be observed, which correlates with the level of consciousness, along with the apparition of characteristic patterns.

To allow a good interpretation, the EEG recording of a patient must last long enough without stimulations to correctly assess the background activity of the EEG and to detect potential variations [3]. It is important to test the reactivity of the EEG to eye opening/closing and external stimulations. A reactive EEG reflects a lighter coma and is associated with a better prognosis [3, 6]. Auditory or nociceptive stimulations can be used. Reactivity can be characterized by a drop in the background activity or by an increase in amplitude. Synek [7] suggested a scale to assess the severity of the coma. This scale has then been adapted by Young et al. in order to improve its reproducibility [6]. Young's scale is presented in Table 6.1 and gives information on the level of the coma. Following a lesion of the brainstem, some comatose patients can display an EEG that is comparable to a normal wake EEG with a predominant alpha rhythm – the alpha coma. In the case of an alpha coma, EEG changes can be observed in response to sensory stimuli and to eye openings [3, 8]. These patients must be differentiated from patients suffering a locked-in syndrome or patients in a psychogenic coma. Indeed, in both the latter cases, the EEG can appear normal [3].

The EEG is useful for detecting a loss of consciousness due to non convulsive epileptic seizures or epileptic spikes in patients that are unconscious for other reasons than epilepsy [5]. A nonconvulsive epileptic seizure does not present the usual signs of a complex partial seizure like oculomotor and masticatory muscles contraction, and the patient can appear confused, drowsy, or comatosed. The EEG will show a continuous epileptic activity. If the patient does not react to administered antiepileptic drugs and if the cause of the seizures cannot be treated, the prognosis will be poor [9]. The EEG can also detect epileptic seizures due to a cerebral lesion. In this case, the seizures can be treated.

In case of a loss of consciousness due to a focal supratentorial cerebral lesion, the EEG is significantly abnormal. Different types of abnormalities can be observed,

Table 6.1 EEG classification introduced by Young and collaborators [6]

Category	Subcategory
1. Delta/theta >50% of record (no theta coma)	(a) Reactivity (b) No reactivity
2. Triphasic waves	
3. Burst-suppression	(a) With epileptiform activity (b) Without epileptiform activity
4. Alpha/theta/spindle coma (unreactive)	
5. Epileptiform activity (no burst-suppression pattern)	(a) Generalized (b) Focal or multifocal
6. Suppression	(a) <20 μV but >10 μV (b) <10 μV

Guidelines:
1. Burst-suppression pattern should present generalized flattening at standard sensitivity for more than 1 s at least every 20 s
2. Suppression: for this category, voltage criteria should be met for the entire recording; there should be no reactivity
3. When more than 1 category is present, select the most critical one

such as polymorphic delta activity or epileptic spikes. Nevertheless, the EEG gives little information about the location of the lesion; it can just hardly determine the damaged hemisphere [3].

The last stage of the coma is characterized by burst suppression, when there is no cerebral activity higher than 2 μV. An inactive EEG that lasts for more than 6 h in a patient who is not in hypothermia suggests prosencephalon death but not necessarily cerebral death as the EEG does not reflect the activity of the brainstem [5]. In some rare occasions, patients in permanent vegetative state can have an inactive EEG [3]. Similarly, drug intoxication can lead to an inactive EEG, but it is often reversible.

The interpretation of an EEG recording does not allow a prognostic statement if it is not combined with the etiology. Indeed, the characteristics features of the EEG are not specific to one etiology. Here are some examples of poor prognosis. In case of a cardiac arrest, a periodic generalized pattern is of poor prognosis. *Following a hypoxia or metabolic encephalopathy, the apparition of suppression periods lasting several seconds that are not followed by a burst are of poor prognosis.* A pattern such as alpha coma or alpha-theta coma is associated with different prognosis based on the etiology. For instance, if it is associated with a brainstem lesion, it is of poor prognosis. For a detailed review of prognosis associated with different patterns, we recommend the article by Brenner [3].

Evoked Potentials

Evoked potentials allow an objective evaluation of patients' sensory and cognitive functions. Changes due to sensory, motor, or cognitive activity are invisible when recording the raw EEG because of low signal-to-noise ratio. To observe them, the stimulus must be repeated several times. Auditory evoked potentials are most often elicited by sounds (clics) presented through headphones. Somato-sensory evoked potentials are elicited by stimulation of the median nerve, near the wrist. Visual evoked potentials elicited by flashes are less common because they do not always trigger a response, even in healthy controls [10]. To observe an evoked potential, the EEG must be windowed around the stimulus, each window having the same size and starting at the same moment with respect to the stimulus. These windows are then averaged and, therefore, activities that systematically arise at the same time interval after the stimulus will add up while other cerebral activity not related to the stimulus will be averaged out. This procedure reveals positive and negative variations in the EEG called "*components*." These components are markers of the activity of cerebral areas related to stimulus processing.

Components obtained in response to a sensory stimulation reflect the processing of the stimulus through time, from low level peripheral receptive structures up to high level associative cerebral areas. The faster components, linked to the physical properties of the stimulus are called "*exogenous*" and reflect the activation of neurons projecting toward the primary cortex. Belated components are linked to the psychological signification of the stimulus, experimental conditions, and the level of awareness. They are called "*endogenous*" components and reflect the activity of subcortical and cortical structures, including associative areas.

Somesthetic-evoked potentials (SEP) are obtained by transcutaneous electric stimulation of median nerves in the wrist. These potentials reflect the conduction of the nervous influx through the brachial plexus and its access to the primary somatosensory cortex [11]. A bilateral absence of the N20 in a comatose patient is highly associated with an absence of consciousness recovery (in 99–100% of cases) [12–15]. Brainstem auditory evoked potentials (BAEP) are useful to study the conduction of the auditory signal via the auditory nerve and the protuberance. They appear within 10 ms. The absence of these potentials is associated with a poor recovery in patients with severe cerebral lesions but without peripheral auditory lesions [16, 17]. Nevertheless, this component has a lower predictive value than the N20 response [13].

The absence of exogenous components is a marker of poor prognosis [18]. Most of the patients for whom these components are bilaterally absent either die or stay in permanent vegetative state. However, the presence of exogenous components is not informative enough to be a marker of good prognosis. Clear exogenous components can be observed in patients that never recover.

More advanced cerebral processes, possibly reflecting the presence of consciousness, can be studied using cognitive-evoked potentials. Until now they were exclusively studied with auditory tasks because comatose patients do not have eye-gaze control. They differ from exogenous-evoked potentials in the sense that they are highly dependent on the experimental conditions. It is, thus, important to record these potentials when the patient is most vigilant and to ensure that the paradigm is optimized for recording the best potentials while minimizing the number of repetitions to avoid a habituation effect. There are five main components usually studied: the N100 component in response to a stimulus, the mismatch negativity and the P3 in response to novelty, and N400 and P600 components in response to semantic changes.

The N100 component, a negative inflection that appears 100 ms after the start of the stimulus, indicates a response of the auditory cortex. This component is elicited by all types of stimuli and reveals that the auditory cortex is properly functioning. Its predictive value is, however, highly debated [19–22]. Aside BAEPs, the N100 component would yet have a lower predictive value than the N20 response as regards consciousness recovery in comatose patients [13].

The mismatch negativity (MMN) is a negative component, which appears between 100 and 200 ms after a change or odd sound following a series of monotonous sounds. This component has low amplitude, which implies that a high number of repetitions are necessary for a good visualization. Since the MMN does not require the subject's attention, it indicates an automatic response triggered by the difference between the dissonant sound and the other preceding sounds which are still recorded in memory. Previous data obtained with an MMN paradigm in comatose patients suggest that this component beholds important predictive value independent of the etiology. Indeed, an absence of this response was related to an absence of recovery in 91–93% of cases [13, 23]. This component, likewise the N20 response, has a better predictive value than AEPCTs or the N100 response [13, 24].

Kotchoubey et al. have shown that the MMN component could be present in minimally conscious patients (34%) and in patients in a vegetative state as well (65%) [25]. However, recently, Wijnen et al. demonstrated that for ten vegetative patients, the amplitude of the MMN was significantly higher in patients who evolved later to a minimally conscious state [26].

The P3 is a positive inflexion generated when the subject detects a rare and unexpected stimulus. For an auditory potential, it appears approximately 300 ms after the stimulus, while for a visual stimulus it can appear 500 or 600 ms after the stimulus presentation. In case of cerebral lesions, its latency can be higher [27, 28]. The MMN and P3 are two different cerebral responses elicited by similar stimuli (deviant or novel), but they differ according to the time interval between stimuli. The MMN is generated when the stimuli are close to one another but disappears when the interval between two stimuli is longer than 2 s. The MMN originates from the superior temporal gyrus and from the frontal cortex. The P3 relates to the activation of a network of cerebral areas including frontoparietal regions [29]. The P3 is frequently linked to cognitive processes of higher complexity than the N100 and MMN components, such as categorization, decision-making, or updates in working memory. If simple sounds are sufficient for the generation of an MMN or a P3, the latter can also be generated by more complex stimuli. The emotional valence of these stimuli will have an impact on the amplitude. A stimulus such as the own name will more likely trigger a P3 than a simple sound [30, 31] (Fig. 6.1). The presence of an MMN and/or a P3 in acute minimally conscious patients is considered as a sign of good prognostic but cannot disentangle patients in a vegetative state from patients in a minimally conscious state [32–35]. From a behavioral viewpoint, the distinction between these two states can be made based on response to command. Hence, active-evoked potentials are used to better evaluate consciousness in a patient as it requires his/her active participation, which differs from passive listening. In an experience where patients were asked to count occurrences of their own name,

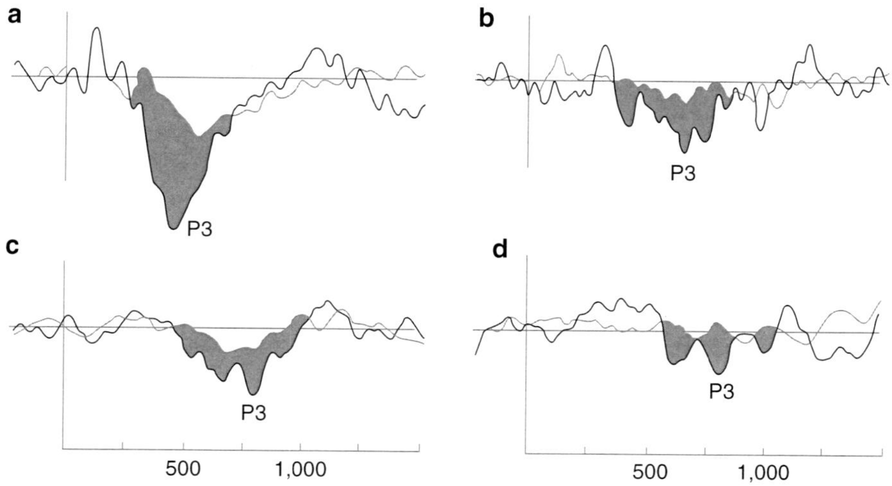

Fig. 6.1 Auditory evoked potentials in response to the own name in (**a**) healthy controls ($n=5$), (**b**) locked in syndrome patients ($n=4$), (**c**) minimally conscious patients ($n=6$) and (**d**) vegetative patients ($n=5$). The area in *grey* represents the difference in activation between the presentation of the own name and the presentation of other names. A P3 response can be observed even in some patients in a vegetative state. Electrode Pz (Adapted from [30])

presented along with seven other names, some minimally conscious patients displayed a P3 of greater amplitude than when passively listening to their name. On the other hand, vegetative patients who showed a P3 in response to their name did not display higher amplitudes when asked to actively count their names [31]. These tasks have a similar goal than active tasks used in fMRI and are presented in another chapter of this book.

The N400 is a negative inflexion which appears roughly 400 ms after a word presentation. Its amplitude is increased if the stimulus is discordant (semantic or phonologic discordances) based on the context (word or sentence). Care must be taken, however, as a semantic incongruence can also lead to a P600, a positive inflexion which appears 600 ms after stimulus presentation. Any change, negative or positive, can, thus, be considered as incongruence processing. These inflexions can also be observed in inattentive healthy controls, and therefore it can be assumed that like the MMN and P3, they result from an automatic process [33].

Evoked potentials are complementary to behavioral studies in patients. They can be used according to a hierarchical approach [36] where low level functionalities are first evaluated with exogenous potentials and then higher level processing is tested with cognitive potentials. The latter is presented in passive and then in active tasks. If the patient answers to the active task, he demonstrates a response to command. At this stage, it becomes important to test communication tools with the patient such as brain–computer interfaces, which are the scope of another chapter included in this book.

Quantitative Electroencephalography

Quantitative electroencephalography (qEEG) consists in the use of algorithms in order to extract complex measures likely to add objective information that cannot be extracted from visual inspection of the EEG traces. For instance, one can compute the power spectral density of the signal at each electrode location, assess the level of connectivity between electrodes, or use measures based on signal complexity as employed in anesthesia to establish the level of consciousness of a patient. Practically, a qEEG analysis consists in the extraction of non artifacted temporal windows, lasting from one to several seconds, from a recordings lasting several minutes. The different required parameters are computed on each of these windows and then averaged in order to provide a global value. Furthermore, building large EEG datasets enable the use of statistical tools allowing a diagnostic or prognostic evaluation of groups of patients.

The power spectral density can be obtained from the fast Fourier transform or a wavelet transform computed on the extracted windows. It is expressed in absolute power (uV^2) or in relative power (%) for each individual electrode or for a subgroup of electrodes corresponding to a region of interest. In comatose patients, the power spectral density is higher in lower frequencies while it is lower in higher frequencies as compared to healthy controls. Such findings can also be observed visually in EEG traces (Fig. 6.2) [37, 38].

Tools initially developed for anesthesia monitoring have been proposed to evaluate the level of consciousness in severely brain-injured patients. These tools are used in the clinical field to measure the depth of anesthesia and to prevent the patient's arousal during a surgical procedure, while allowing drug savings and a faster postoperative awakening thanks to a better control of the depth of anesthesia.

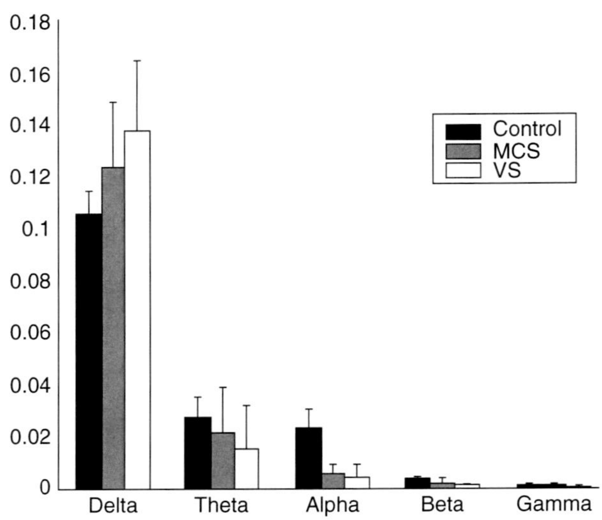

Fig. 6.2 Normalized power spectral density computed at Cz in five different frequency bands in healthy controls ($n = 5$), patients in a minimally conscious state ($n = 12$, MCS) and patients in a vegetative state ($n = 10$, VS). Patients have more power in low frequency bands and less power in higher frequency bands

Furthermore they are easy to use and interpret. For example, the bispectral index (BIS) is a unitless measure ranging from 0 (inactive EEG) to 100 (normal activity), which results from a combination of temporal and frequency parameters [39]. During sleep, BIS values gradually decrease [40]. In case of disorders of consciousness, vegetative patients have a lower BIS value than patients in a minimally conscious state, but this value cannot systematically differentiate patients in a vegetative state from patients in a minimally conscious state at an individual level [41]. Similar results were obtained using the spectral entropy (EEG-entropy) [42, 43].

The EEG can also help to quantify connectivity between cerebral areas [44]. Connectivity is disrupted in patients suffering from disorders of consciousness [45]. Computing the coupling between electrodes provides a connectivity measure of underlying brain areas. This measure gives complementary information that can be used for diagnostic and prognostic purposes. To correctly interpret this measure, it is important to take into account two inherent limitations: the volume conduction problem and the choice of the reference. Indeed, the reference induces a common component to the signals at each electrode location which will, therefore, appear artificially coupled. It is, thus, advised to use bipolar montages in connectivity studies. Similarly, the diffusion of electrical currents through the cerebrospinal fluid and the bone will result in the fact that different electrodes will record redundant information and, again, will appear artificially connected. Correlation methods and coherence, the spectral equivalent of correlation, are subject to these drawbacks. They can nonetheless provide information, but their interpretation must take into account the reference and volume conduction problem. A study on a single patient in a vegetative state with a damaged right hemisphere showed a diminution of the connectivity in the right hemisphere. Such decrease was not visible using spectral power measures [46]. A coherence decrease has also been observed in minimally conscious patients [47, 48]. Other measures of connectivity have been proposed in the past 10 years to answer the volume conduction problem [44, 49]. The first results with some of these new methods also tend to show a drop of connectivity [38, 48].

Finally, qEEG may also include source reconstruction methods, which estimate the potential brain areas where the electrical signal is coming from [50]. These methods are based on approximations of the brain structure. A core approximation will model the brain as three concentric spheres and a finer approximation will use magnetic resonance images of the patient's brain in order to obtain a realistic model of the brain. All the parameters computed at the scalp level can also be computed at the source level, which provides a better spatial resolution and allows a three dimension visualization of the brain's activity. However, these methods require at least 32 electrodes, 64 or more electrodes being recommended [50].

To conclude, qEEG allows various objective measurements of the cerebral activity providing information on the patient's consciousness level. Encouraging results have shown differences between groups of patients according to the diagnosis and the prognosis. It is, however, not yet possible to target one single parameter allowing an accurate diagnosis at the individual level. Future challenges consist in linking the excellent temporal resolution of the EEG with the spatial resolution of the fMRI in order to have a better comprehension of disorders of consciousness.

Conclusion

While the interpretation of the EEG trace can give some information on the patient's consciousness level and detect epileptic activity, exogenous-evoked potentials can give useful information as regards the patient's prognosis (e.g., N20 or MMN) and remnant stimulus processing. Active cognitive evoked potentials can also detect signs of consciousness such as response to command. Finally, quantitative measures offer a new interpretation of the EEG and provide new objective information (e.g., by using coherence and source reconstruction methods). They, nevertheless, require more testing and improvements before being applied in clinical settings.

References

1. Guideline seven: a proposal for standard montages to be used in clinical EEG. American Electroencephalographic Society. J Clin Neurophysiol. 1994;11:30–6. (http://www.ncbi.nlm.nih.gov/pubmed/8195414)
2. Krauss GL, Fisher RS, editors. The Johns Hopkins atlas of digital EEG: an interactive training guide. Baltimore: The Johns Hopkins University Press; 2006.
3. Brenner RP. The interpretation of the EEG in stupor and coma. Neurologist. 2005;11:271–84.
4. Young GB, et al. Initial assessment and management of the patient with impaired alertness. In: Young GB, editor. Coma and impaired consciousness. New York: McGraw-Hill; 1998. p. 97–103.
5. Posner JB, Saper CB, Schiff ND, Plum F. Plum and Posner's diagnosis of stupor and coma. New York: Oxford University Press; 2007.
6. Young GB, McLachlan RS, Kreeft JH, Demelo JD. An electroencephalographic classification for coma. Can J Neurol Sci. 1997;24:320–5.
7. Synek VM. Prognostically important EEG coma patterns in diffuse anoxic and traumatic encephalopathies in adults. J Clin Neurophysiol. 1988;5:161–74.
8. Westmoreland BF, Klass DW, Sharbrough FW, Reagan TJ. Alpha-coma. Electroencephalographic, clinical, pathologic, and etiologic correlations. Arch Neurol. 1975;32:713–8.
9. Kaplan PW. The clinical features, diagnosis, and prognosis of nonconvulsive status epilepticus. Neurologist. 2005;11:348–61.
10. Vanhaudenhuyse A, Laureys S, Perrin F. Cognitive event-related potentials in comatose and post-comatose states. Neurocrit Care. 2007;8:262–70.
11. Guerit JM. Evoked potentials in severe brain injury. Prog Brain Res. 2005;150:415–26.
12. Amantini A, Grippo A, Fossi S, et al. Prediction of 'awakening' and outcome in prolonged acute coma from severe traumatic brain injury: evidence for validity of short latency SEPs. Clin Neurophysiol. 2005;116:229–35.
13. Fischer C, Luaute J, Nemoz C, et al. Improved prediction of awakening or nonawakening from severe anoxic coma using tree-based classification analysis. Crit Care Med. 2006;34:1520–4.
14. Lew HL, Dikmen S, Slimp J, et al. Use of somatosensory-evoked potentials and cognitive event-related potentials in predicting outcomes of patients with severe traumatic brain injury. Am J Phys Med Rehabil. 2003;82:53–61; quiz 62–4, 80.
15. Robinson LR, Micklesen PJ, Tirschwell DL, Lew HL. Predictive value of somatosensory evoked potentials for awakening from coma. Crit Care Med. 2003;31:960–7.
16. de Sousa LC, Colli BO, Piza MR, et al. Auditory brainstem response: prognostic value in patients with a score of 3 on the Glasgow Coma Scale. Otol Neurotol. 2007;28:426–8.
17. Haupt WF, Pawlik G, Thiel A. Initial and serial evoked potentials in cerebrovascular critical care patients. J Clin Neurophysiol. 2006;23:389–94.

18. Laureys S, Perrin F, Schnakers C, et al. Residual cognitive function in comatose, vegetative and minimally conscious states. Curr Opin Neurol. 2005;18:726–33.
19. Fischer C, Luaute J, Adeleine P, Morlet D. Predictive value of sensory and cognitive evoked potentials for awakening from coma. Neurology. 2004;63:669–73.
20. Glass I, Sazbon L, Groswasser Z. Mapping "cognitive" event-related potentials in prolonged postcoma unawareness state. Clin Electroencephalogr. 1998;29:19–30.
21. Guerit JM, Verougstraete D, de Tourtchaninoff M, et al. ERPs obtained with the auditory oddball paradigm in coma and altered states of consciousness: clinical relationships, prognostic value, and origin of components. Clin Neurophysiol. 1999;110:1260–9.
22. Mutschler V, Chaumeil CG, Marcoux L, et al. Auditory P300 in subjects in a post-anoxic coma. Preliminary data. Neurophysiol Clin. 1996;26:158–63.
23. Naccache L, Puybasset L, Gaillard R, et al. Auditory mismatch negativity is a good predictor of awakening in comatose patients: a fast and reliable procedure. Clin Neurophysiol. 2005;116:988–9.
24. Daltrozzo J, Wioland N, Mutschler V, Kotchoubey B. Predicting coma and other low responsive patients outcome using event-related brain potentials: a meta-analysis. Clin Neurophysiol. 2007;118:606–14.
25. Kotchoubey B, Lang S, Mezger G, et al. Information processing in severe disorders of consciousness: vegetative state and minimally conscious state. Clin Neurophysiol. 2005;116:2441–53.
26. Wijnen VJ, van Boxtel GJ, Eilander HJ, de Gelder B. Mismatch negativity predicts recovery from the vegetative state. Clin Neurophysiol. 2007;118:597–605.
27. Munte TF, Heinze HJ. Brain potentials reveal deficits of language processing after closed head injury. Arch Neurol. 1994;51:482–93.
28. Granovsky Y, Sprecher E, Hemli J, Yarnitsky D. P300 and stress in mild head injury patients. Electroencephalogr Clin Neurophysiol. 1998;108:554–9.
29. Pegado F, Bekinschtein T, Chausson N, et al. Probing the lifetimes of auditory novelty detection processes. Neuropsychologia. 2010;48:3145–54.
30. Perrin F, Schnakers C, Schabus M, et al. Brain response to one's own name in vegetative state, minimally conscious state, and locked-in syndrome. Arch Neurol. 2006;63:562–9.
31. Schnakers C, Perrin F, Schabus M, et al. Voluntary brain processing in disorders of consciousness. Neurology. 2008;71:1614–20.
32. Fischer C, Dailler F, Morlet D. Novelty P3 elicited by the subject's own name in comatose patients. Clin Neurophysiol. 2008;119:2224–30.
33. Vanhaudenhuyse A, Laureys S, Perrin F. Cognitive event-related potentials in comatose and post-comatose states. Neurocrit Care. 2008;8:262–70.
34. Kotchoubey B. Event-related potential measures of consciousness: two equations with three unknowns. Prog Brain Res. 2005;150:427–44.
35. Fischer C, Luaute J, Morlet D. Event-related potentials (MMN and novelty P3) in permanent vegetative or minimally conscious states. Clin Neurophysiol. 2010;121:1032–42.
36. Kubler A, Kotchoubey B. Brain-computer interfaces in the continuum of consciousness. Curr Opin Neurol. 2007;20:643–9.
37. Leon-Carrion J, Martin-Rodriguez JF, Damas-Lopez J, et al. Brain function in the minimally conscious state: a quantitative neurophysiological study. Clin Neurophysiol. 2008;119:1506–14.
38. Lehembre R, Bruno MA, Vanhaudenhuyse A, et al. Resting state EEG study of comatose patients: a connectivity and frequency analysis to find differences between vegetative and minimally conscious states. Funct Neurol 2012 (in press).
39. Johansen JW, Sebel PS. Development and clinical application of electroencephalographic bispectrum monitoring. Anesthesiology. 2000;93:1336–44.
40. Noirhomme Q, Boly M, Bonhomme V, et al. Bispectral index correlates with regional cerebral blood flow during sleep in distinct cortical and subcortical structures in humans. Arch Ital Biol. 2009;147:51–7.
41. Schnakers C, Ledoux D, Majerus S, et al. Diagnostic and prognostic use of bispectral index in coma, vegetative state and related disorders. Brain Inj. 2008;22:926–31.

42. Gosseries O, Schnakers C, Ledoux D, et al. Automated EEG entropy measurements in coma, vegetative state/unresponsive wakefulness syndrome and minimally conscious state. Funct Neurol. 2011;26(1):25–30.
43. Viertio-Oja H, Maja V, Sarkela M, et al. Description of the entropy algorithm as applied in the datex-ohmeda S/5 entropy module. Acta Anaesthesiol Scand. 2004;48:154–61.
44. Pereda E, Quiroga RQ, Bhattacharya J. Nonlinear multivariate analysis of neurophysiological signals. Prog Neurobiol. 2005;77:1–37.
45. Laureys S. The neural correlate of (un)awareness: lessons from the vegetative state. Trends Cogn Sci. 2005;9:556–9.
46. Davey MP, Victor JD, Schiff ND. Power spectra and coherence in the EEG of a vegetative patient with severe asymmetric brain damage. Clin Neurophysiol. 2000;111:1949–54.
47. Schiff N. Large scale brain dynamics and connectivity in the minimally conscious state. In: Handbook of brain connectivity. New York: Springer; 2007. p. 505–20.
48. Pollonini L, Pophale S, Situ N, et al. Information communication networks in severe traumatic brain injury. Brain Topogr. 2010;23:221–6.
49. Stam CJ. Nonlinear dynamical analysis of EEG and MEG: review of an emerging field. Clin Neurophysiol. 2005;116:2266–301.
50. Michel CM, Murray MM, Lantz G, et al. EEG source imaging. Clin Neurophysiol. 2004;115:2195–222.

Chapter 7
Brain-Computer Interface: A Communication Aid?

Camille Chatelle, Zulay Lugo, Quentin Noirhomme, Bettina Sorger, and Dorothee Lulé

Introduction

A brain-computer interface (BCI) is a system allowing for communication between the brain and the external environment. It is independent from any peripheral neural or muscular activity and it directly converts brain activity into a computerized command [1]. A BCI is based on cerebral activity measured using techniques, such as electroencephalography (EEG), functional magnetic resonance imagery (fMRI),

C. Chatelle, M.Sc. (✉) • Q. Noirhomme, Ph.D.
Coma Science Group, Cyclotron Research Center, University of Liège,
Allée du Six août, 8, 4000 Liège, Belgium
e-mail: camille.chatelle@ulg.ac.be; quentin.noirhomme@ulg.ac.be

Z. Lugo, M.Sc.
Coma Science Group, Cyclotron Research Center, University of Liège,
Allée du Six août, 8, 4000 Liège, Belgium

Department of Psychology I, Biological Psychology, Clinical Psychology and Psychotherapy, University of Würzburg, Würzburg, Germany
e-mail: zrlugo@yahoo.com

B. Sorger, Ph.D.
Coma Science Group, Cyclotron Research Center, University of Liège,
Allée du Six août, 8, 4000 Liège, Belgium

Department of Cognitive Neuroscience, Faculty of Psychology and Neuroscience, Maastricht University and Maastricht Brain Imaging Centre (M-BIC), Maastricht, The Netherlands
e-mail: b.sorger@maastrichtuniversity.nl

D. Lulé, Ph.D.
Section of Neurophysiology, Department of Neurology, University of Ulm,
Albert-Einstein-Allee 47, Ulm, Germany
e-mail: dorothee.lule@uni-ulm.de

C. Schnakers, S. Laureys (eds.), *Coma and Disorders of Consciousness*,
DOI 10.1007/978-1-4471-2440-5_7, © Springer-Verlag London 2012

implanted electrodes or functional near-infrared spectroscopy (fNIRS) in order to control the environment [2]. A BCI is not a "mind-reading" device. Its primary function is to provide the subject a virtual keyboard, whose keys are pressed using brain activity. Each key press constitutes a choice of an item from a set of items. This choice is made through the control of neuroelectrical activity [3–5]. A specific algorithm translates the extracted features into commands that represent the users' intent. These commands can control effectors to select items (e.g., words). Recent development has shown the usefulness of BCIs in controlling motor prosthesis, cursors, access to internet, and communication [5–10]. Here, we focused on systems allowing functional communication with the surrounding. These tools, extensively validated in healthy volunteers, could be of interest particularly for communicating with patients whose cognitive functions are intact but are paralyzed and anarthric following a neurological or muscular damage, e.g., patients with a locked-in syndrome (LIS) [11]. Several methods have been developed to allow communication with these patients. The simplest is based on eye movements or blinks [e.g., one eye blink for *yes*, two blinks for *no*]. There are other methods allowing the expression of more complex ideas using alphabetic systems [12]. These methods are based on the patient's residual motor ability. However, in some cases, it is necessary to use a communication system that does not involve motor skills at all. Those motor-independent systems are not only useful for using alphabetic systems and expressing more complex ideas [12]. BCIs could be the key to providing access to the outside world for a LIS patient [13]. Finally, beyond communication, it is also possible to use these systems as a diagnostic aid in patients with disorders of consciousness (DOC). In fact, it could be used to detect a response to a command in the absence of discernible behavior at the bedside [14]. Here, we present the recent progress in the development of BCIs. Moreover, we discuss clinical applications in LIS patients and studies performed in patients recovering from coma.

BCI Techniques

Electroencephalography – EEG

BCIs based on EEG use evoked potentials (ERPs), more precisely components such as the P3 or steady-state visually evoked potentials (SSVEPs), sensorimotor rhythms (SMRs), slow cortical potentials (SCPs) and the alpha rhythm. The use of ERPs is a common approach in BCI research. The most widely used component is the P3, a positive deflection occurring about 300 ms after the presentation of a target stimulus. The advantage of using P3 BCIs is that these may include up to 36 different commands. Donchin and his colleagues have developed a visual BCI using a 6×6 matrix composed of letters and signs [15]. The rows and columns are successively illuminated. The subject has to focus his/her attention on the letter he/she wants to spell, eliciting a P3. With this type of BCI, users would be able to spell up to 7–8

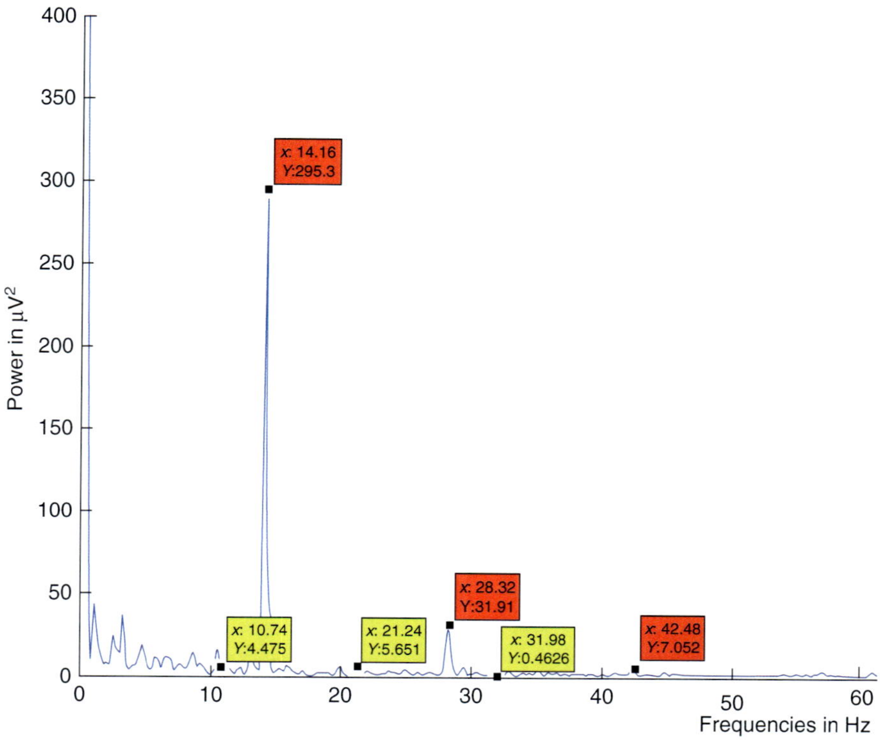

Fig. 7.1 SSVEP. Electrical brain responses (fast Fourier transformed) observed in response to two visual stimuli flashing at a frequency of 10 (*yellow*) and 14 Hz (*red*). The subject had to focus on the 14 Hz stimulus. Here, the first three harmonics in response to these stimuli are represented (Illustration by Nicolas Partoune)

letters per minute with an accuracy of 80–90%. This paradigm has also been adapted to the auditory modality, although the performance achieved is lower and the system has been reported as requiring higher concentration [16]. Those nonvisual P3-based BCIs have been developed for patients who lost control of their eye movements or who are blind [3, 16–18]. Sellers and Donchin [3] tested a BCI for binary communication. In this paradigm, the user hears a sequence of four stimuli (yes, no, stop, go) presented in randomized order. He/she should, then, focus on either *yes* or *no* in each sequence. The task required to count the number of times the target (either *yes* or *no*) was presented. The probability of the selected target stimulus was 0.25, which is sufficient to elicit a P3 [15]. The authors have shown a reliable response during ten sessions in healthy volunteers. Halder also showed the reliability of an auditory BCI for binary communication [19], with an efficiency of 2.46 bits/min and a classification accuracy of 78.5%. Some researchers have focused on other components of ERPs such as the SSVEPs. These are visual ERPs and are elicited in occipital and parieto-occipital areas in response to visual stimulation. These are of small amplitude, consistent [20] (Fig. 7.1) and not susceptible to be influenced by ocular and electromyographic artefacts [21]. The SSVEP-based BCIs offer the possibility of using 2–13 different commands without affecting the classification accuracy (64–96.5%) [21]. Those BCIs have shown their reliability with respect to the control of a cursor to execute commands or to control prosthesis [21]. A recent study has shown its applicability for communication using a spelling words system based on letters flashing at different frequencies [22]. The authors reported an average accuracy of 92.25% and an efficiency of 37.62 bits/min (or 5.51 letters/min).

Changes in SMRs or μ rhythms have also been used for BCI purposes. SMRs refer to EEG activity of 8–15 Hz that can be recorded in primary sensorimotor areas [1] and which is usually accompanied by a beta activity (18–26 Hz). This activity can be reduced or desynchronized by preparing, executing, or imagining a movement (event-related desynchronization), particularly in the contralateral motor region. An increase in the SMR, or synchronization, occurs following the execution of a movement and during relaxation [23]. The advantage here is that these components do not require the actual execution of the movement but solely the kinaesthetic mental imagery of this [24]. However, it is not possible to use more than two commands, the increase to three or more leading to a decrease in the classification accuracy. In healthy subjects, many BCIs have shown satisfying results in producing words based on visual [25] and auditory [26] input. The lowest frequencies of signals generated by the cortex and recorded at the scalp are the SCPs. The negative SCPs are usually associated with movements and other functions that involve cortical activation, while positive SCPs are usually associated with a reduction in cortical activity [27]. This system is also limited to two (or less) commands. It has been shown that it is possible to teach participants to control their brain activity (i.e., the SCPs) to move an object on a screen [28]. In this context, communication systems have been developed for patients with LIS (see below).

Alpha rhythms have also been implemented for BCIs. Vidal was the first to show that it was possible to determine the position of eye gaze and the direction in which the user wants to move a cursor through the activity generated in the visual cortex [29]. Implicit changes in visual attention are associated with a desynchronization in alpha rhythm in the posterior regions, contralateral [30] to the target position and with an ipsilateral synchronization [31]. A BCI was then developed by van Gerven and colleagues [32] based on implicit spatial attention. They showed the possibility of using the alpha band power to classify subjects' responses ($n = 15$) with an accuracy of 29–69% (25% chance level). This paradigm has also shown a rate of 20 bits/min.

Neuroimaging

Even though it is more expensive than EEG, fMRI is also a technique used for BCIs, especially due to its high spatial resolution. It measures changes in the blood oxygenation level in the brain (hemodynamic activity) and is related to neuronal activity [33]. Boly and colleagues proposed a paradigm based on motor and visual imagery (i.e., to imagine *playing tennis* versus to *imagine visiting the own house*). Both tasks showed clearly distinct brain activation in the supplementary motor and parahippocampal areas, respectively [34]. To establish a communication, Monti and colleagues asked participants to respond to autobiographical questions by *yes* or *no* using one of these mental imagery tasks. At the end of each sequence (5 min), the researchers were able to infer the responses of 16 participants with an accuracy of 100% [35]. Recently, another paradigm has been proposed to allow more complex communication than binary yes/no answers. Sorger and colleagues [2] have tested a communication paradigm in eight healthy volunteers using two mental tasks (e.g., motor imagery and mental arithmetic) and different temporal answer parameters (task onset and duration). The questions were related to multiple choice answers (A, B, C, or D). For answering a question, the participants had to look at the letter corresponding to the target response and perform the mental task associated to this letter as long as this one was illuminated on the screen (Fig. 7.2). Across all participants, 37 out of 39 responses were correctly decoded (94.7%). In six participants, the accuracy was of 100%, and in the other two participants, it remained above the level of chance (85.7% and 75%, chance level being 25%).

Another promising BCI technique is fNIRS. Like fMRI, it measures the hemodynamic response of the brain [36]. The main advantage of the fNIRS as opposed to fMRI is that it is portable and less sensitive to motion artefacts. However, it measures activity in the cortex, and cannot reach deep areas (more than 3 cm deep) in contrast to fMRI. Coyle and colleagues have proposed a BCI (*Mindswitch*) based on one channel allowing generating two commands (*yes/no*) and then offering a binary communication [37]. Several studies have also shown the usefulness of the fNIRS-based BCIs using multiple channels [38, 39] and reporting accuracy between 80% and 89% in healthy subjects (50% chance level).

Development of BCIs as Diagnostic and Communication Tools in DOC

EEG-Based BCIs

EEG-based BCIs have been applied in patients with amyotrophic lateral sclerosis (ALS) [5, 40]. However, there is variability in the results. One study showed that it was possible to establish communication [40] in five out of six ALS patients using the P3-based paradigm developed by Donchin [15]. Four of them used this system later for spelling words and have demonstrated functional communication. Sellers and Donchin showed reliable responses in ALS patients with their auditory paradigm based on four stimuli (yes, no, stop, go), despite lower accuracies than in healthy participants [3]. Kübler has adapted the use of a matrix in the auditory modality. Five rows and five columns represented the letters of the alphabet [17]. The five lines were associated with a number between 1 and 5 and the five columns

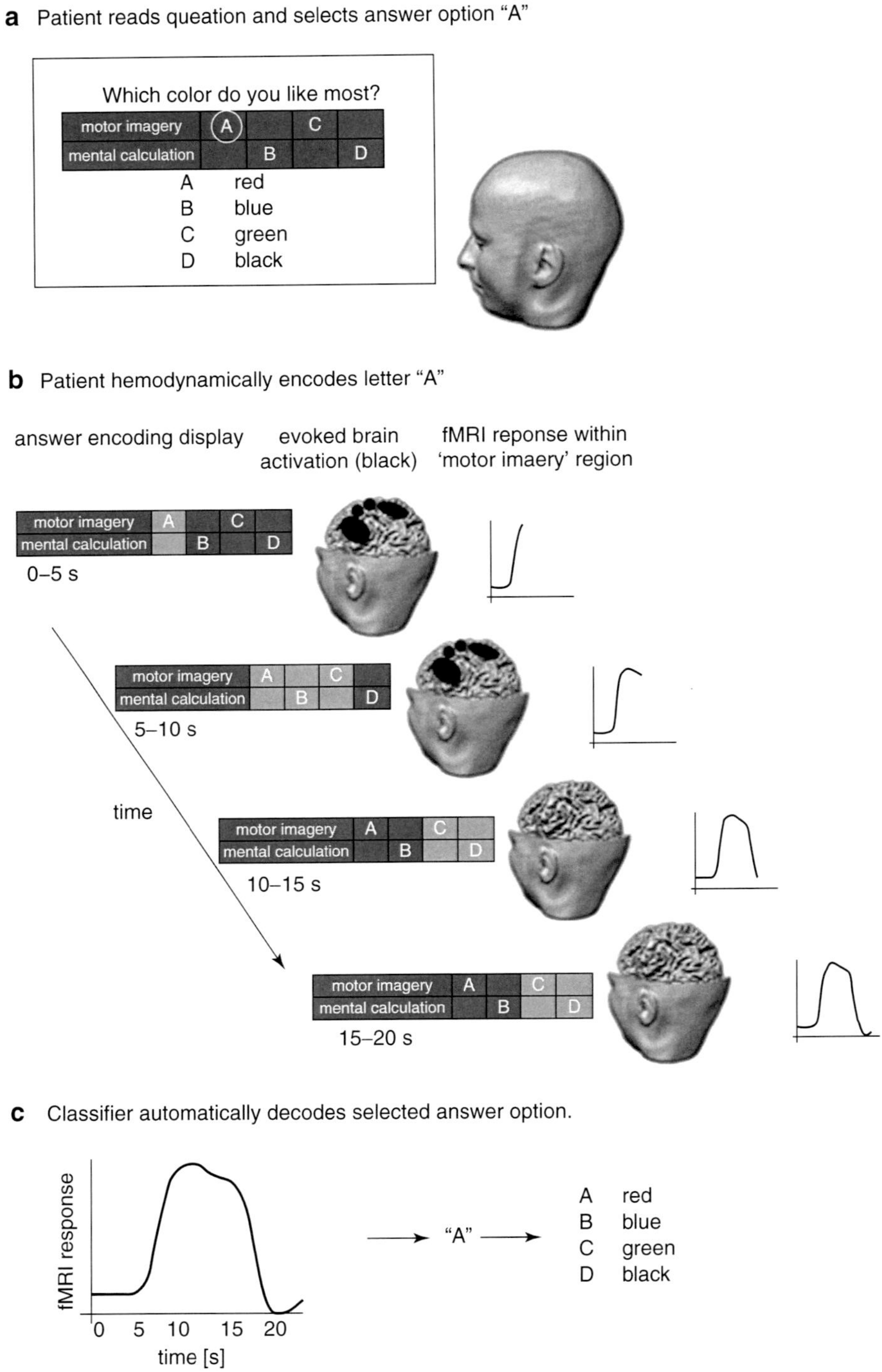
a Patient reads queation and selects answer option "A"
Which color do you like most?
motor imagery
mental calculation
A
B
C
D
A red
B blue
C green
D black
b Patient hemodynamically encodes letter "A"
answer encoding display
evoked brain activation (black)
fMRI reponse within 'motor imaery' region
0–5 s
5–10 s
10–15 s
15–20 s
time
c Classifier automatically decodes selected answer option.
fMRI response
0 5 10 15 20
time [s]
"A"
A red
B blue
C green
D black

with a number between 6 and 10. The numbers were auditorily presented and the patient selected the row and the column of the target letter. Four ALS patients were evaluated with this system, demonstrating adequate performance for visual (more than 70%) but not for auditory (just above chance level) communication. Moreover, users reported more difficulty to concentrate in the auditory condition. To our knowledge, Lulé and colleagues performed the first study in patients with DOC [41]. They used the Sellers and Donchin's paradigm to test its reliability as a diagnostic tool. The results have shown its benefits in improving the detection of consciousness in patients with DOC (Fig. 7.3). Two LIS patients were also evaluated, only one of them having reliably used the BCI. This shows that the system cannot ensure the absence of consciousness in case of negative results [41].

Using SMRs, Neuper and colleagues [43] have trained a paralyzed patient to use a language support program (LSP, [44]) in order to communicate. The spelling involved the selection of a letter in successive steps using a virtual keyboard. A predefined set of letters was divided in two subsets and presented at the top and at the bottom of the screen. The patient was instructed to select one of this subset by either relaxing or by using motor imagery. When the patient had selected the subset containing the target letter, this subset was itself divided into two parts, and this until the patient selected the target letter. After several months, the patient was able to control the keyboard with an accuracy of 70%. Another study showed the possibility for a patient with ALS to use a keyboard by the control of SMRs [45]. These evoked potentials were also recently used with DOC patients. Cruse and colleagues have detected command following (i.e., *to imagine squeezing the right hand* versus *to imagine moving all the fingers or toes*) in a patient clinically diagnosed as being in a vegetative state [46]. As with SMRs, the LSP can be used by patients via the control of SCPs rhythms [47, 48]. Patients with advanced ALS showed their abilities, after training, to use the LSP in increasing or decreasing their brain activity to select the block corresponding to the target letter and then to write words [42].

Fig. 7.2 Answering multiple-choice questions based on intentionally generated single-trial fMRI responses (example). (*Panel* **a**) A question and four answer options are displayed on a screen. The participant is asked to select an answer and identify the corresponding letter in a letter encoding display (see *gray table*). In the present example, the patient selects letter "A" (located in first row and second column in the table; see *white circle*). (*Panel* **b**) During answer encoding, the patient performs the specific mental task that is shown in the same row as the desired letter ("motor imagery", in the present example). The patient performs this task as long as the desired letter is highlighted by a light gray bar that moves from the left to the right side of the display during each answer encoding trial. In the present example, in order to encode the letter *A*, the patient has to perform "motor imagery" for the first 10 s of the trial. The patient's performance results in a specific spatiotemporal pattern of brain activation, which, in the present example, is unique to the letter *A* (see brain activations in *right column*). (*Panel* **c**) During answer decoding, an algorithm classifies the patient's answer using multifilter correlations. More specifically, the obtained brain activation pattern (in the present example, within a "motor imagery" region) is compared to four different template patterns, with each template corresponding to one of the four possible answers. In this way, the patient's answer is decoded fully automatically and immediately after each trial (i.e., answer)

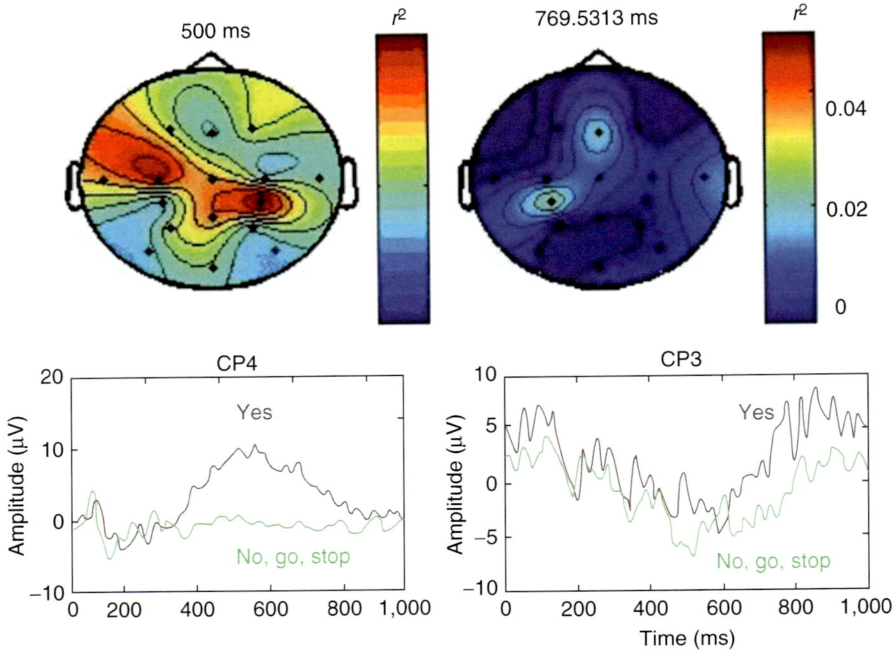

Fig. 7.3 P3 in a healthy volunteer (*left*) and a patient in a minimally conscious state (*right*) in response to the target stimulus *yes*. On the *top*, distribution of the observed response to target stimuli can be seen (yes). The colors in the images in the upper row represent the difference in the observed response between the target stimuli and nontarget stimuli. The greater the difference, the more the region is colored *red–orange*. Below, averaging over all responses for the other three stimuli (nontargets no, stop, go; in *green*) and for all responses to target stimuli (yes; in *brown*) is shown (Adapted from [42])

fMRI-Based BCIs

Functional MRI is particularly useful for the diagnosis of DOC rather than for communication in LIS patients. The paradigm of mental imagery developed by Boly and colleagues [34] was administered to a patient diagnosed as being in a vegetative state. When she was asked to *imagine playing tennis* and *visiting her house*, the patient showed an activity similar to controls on both tasks in the supplementary motor areas and parahippocampal regions, suggesting she understood and followed the command [14]. A few months later, she evolved into a minimally conscious state. This case illustrates the importance of alternative techniques in the diagnosis of patients recovering from coma. In fact, it appears that the patient was at that time unable to show signs of consciousness through any other technique. Subsequently, 54 patients were studied using this protocol and five of them showed a response similar to controls (four being diagnosed in a vegetative state and one in a minimally conscious state) [49]. A *yes/no* communication was established in one of these patients using fMRI. The patient was able to adequately respond five out of six questions using mental imagery tasks, supporting the usefulness of this technique in establishing a functional communication in patients unable to communicate at the bedside.

The fNIRS is a fairly new technique that has not been much studied in BCI research. To our knowledge, there is only one study demonstrating the usefulness of fNIRS as a communication tool for patients. Naito and colleagues used fNIRS in 40 ALS patients, including 17 total LIS [50]. They used a single channel and two wavelengths (770 and 840 nm) measuring the activity in the frontal area. The subjects had to answer various questions with a "*yes*" by performing mental arithmetic or singing (and, hence, increasing their brain activity in frontal regions), or a "*no*" by relaxing. The results show that 70% of incomplete LIS patients and 40% of patients with a complete LIS were able to respond *yes/no* with an accuracy of 80%.

Invasive BCIs Systems

So far, we have presented BCIs using noninvasive systems. As many systems are based on EEG signals measured on the scalp, the quality of recordings is relatively low (distorted signal and low amplitude), the spatial resolution is limited and training is necessary. Therefore, some studies have focused on invasive recording methods. Recordings are performed either directly at the neuronal level [51, 52] or on the brain surface in the case of an electrocorticographic recording [53–55]. BCIs based on intracortical microelectrodes can directly record the activity of neurons and provide a stronger signal. These allow users to control devices such as computer cursors more quickly and accurately [55]. While this technique has not been tested in healthy subjects, patients showed good performances in the context of complex communication (spelling words) [52, 54]. This technique, nevertheless, implies clinical risks and its reliability is limited. Therefore, there is still a long way to go before this device could be used in LIS patients on a daily basis [1].

Conclusion and Perspectives

We have presented a review of the literature on various BCIs tested in patients with severe motor disabilities. The success in using a BCI still varies considerably between individuals. If some systems work in healthy subjects, this does not necessarily mean that it will work in specific patient-target groups, e.g., in severely paralyzed patients [56]. In about 20% of potential users, the accuracy obtained is not sufficient to allow the patient to control an application [57]. Therefore, it seems important to validate BCIs directly in the target population and to adapt these to the needs and the problems specific to this population (e.g., to use auditory paradigms if visual control problems occur). In the future, it is important to develop systems that are reliable and easy to use in the everyday life. New algorithms should include the automatic detection of artefacts, single-trial classification, and the possibility to classify a session without training sessions.

BCIs might provide useful information about patients recovering from coma. These could be used to improve the clinical diagnosis as it has already been suggested by fMRI and EEG studies using imagery tasks. However, the typical vigilance fluctuation observed in DOC patients is a major confounding factor for this BCI application [58]. Indeed, fMRI could demonstrate reliable detection of signs of consciousness in patients diagnosed as being in a vegetative state. However, many patients have been evaluated and only a few have shown signs of consciousness with this paradigm, including patients showing signs of consciousness at the bedside. Further research is needed to know whether this is due to a lack of awareness in some patients, or due to vigilance fluctuation. Currently available BCI systems will have to be tested in such patients. Active tasks such as motor imagery seem to be promising in the detection of signs of consciousness [2, 13, 14, 16, 19, 34, 40].

References

1. Wolpaw JR, Birbaumer N, McFarland DJ, et al. Brain-computer interfaces for communication and control. Clin Neurophysiol. 2002;113(6):767–91.
2. Sorger B, Dahmen B, Reithler J, et al. Another kind of 'BOLD Response': answering multiple-choice questions via online decoded single-trial brain signals. Prog Brain Res. 2009;177: 275–92.
3. Sellers EW, Donchin E. A P300-based brain-computer interface: initial tests by ALS patients. Clin Neurophysiol. 2006;117(3):538–48.
4. Sellers EW, Kubler A, Donchin E. Brain-computer interface research at the University of South Florida Cognitive Psychophysiology Laboratory: the P300 speller. IEEE Trans Neural Syst Rehabil Eng. 2006;14(2):221–4.
5. Kübler A. Brain-computer interfaces for communication in paralysed patients and implications for disorders of consciousness. In: Laureys S, Tononi G, editors. The neurology of consciousness. London/Burlington/San Diego: Academic Press/Elsevier; 2008. p. 217–34.
6. Citi L, Poli R, Cinel C, Sepulveda F. P300-based BCI mouse with genetically-optimized analogue control. IEEE Trans Neural Syst Rehabil Eng. 2008;16(1):51–61.
7. Yoo SS, Fairneny T, Chen NK, et al. Brain-computer interface using fMRI: spatial navigation by thoughts. Neuroreport. 2004;15(10):1591–5.
8. Mugler EM, Ruf CA, Halder S, et al. Design and implementation of a P300-based brain-computer interface for controlling an internet browser. IEEE Trans Neural Syst Rehabil Eng. 2010;18:599–609.
9. Sellers EW, Vaughan TM, Wolpaw JR. A brain-computer interface for long-term independent home use. Amyotroph Lateral Scler. 2010;11:449–55.
10. Lee JH, Ryu J, Jolesz FA, et al. Brain-machine interface via real-time fMRI: preliminary study on thought-controlled robotic arm. Neurosci Lett. 2009;450(1):1–6.
11. Schnakers C, Majerus S, Goldman S, et al. Cognitive function in the locked-in syndrome. J Neurol. 2008;255(3):323–30.
12. Bruno MA, Schnakers C, Damas F, et al. Locked-in syndrome in children: report of five cases and review of the literature. Pediatr Neurol. 2009;41(4):237–46.
13. Kubler A, Neumann N. Brain-computer interfaces–the key for the conscious brain locked into a paralyzed body. Prog Brain Res. 2005;150:513–25.

14. Owen AM, Coleman MR, Boly M, et al. Detecting awareness in the vegetative state. Science. 2006;313(5792):1402.
15. Donchin E, Spencer KM, Wijesinghe R. The mental prosthesis: assessing the speed of a P300-based brain-computer interface. IEEE Trans Rehabil Eng. 2000;8(2):174–9.
16. Furdea A, Halder S, Krusienski DJ, et al. An auditory oddball (P300) spelling system for brain-computer interfaces. Psychophysiology. 2009;46(3):617–25.
17. Kubler A, Furdea A, Halder S, et al. A brain-computer interface controlled auditory event-related potential (p300) spelling system for locked-in patients. Ann N Y Acad Sci. 2009; 1157:90–100.
18. Schreuder M, Blankertz B, Tangermann M. A new auditory multi-class brain-computer interface paradigm: spatial hearing as an informative cue. PLoS One. 2010;5(4):e9813.
19. Halder S, Rea M, Andreoni R, et al. An auditory oddball brain-computer interface for binary choices. Clin Neurophysiol. 2010;121(4):516–23.
20. Regan D. Some characteristics of average steady-state and transient responses evoked by modulated light. Electroencephalogr Clin Neurophysiol. 1966;20(3):238–48.
21. Vialatte FB, Maurice M, Dauwels J, Cichocki A. Steady-state visually evoked potentials: focus on essential paradigms and future perspectives. Prog Neurobiol. 2010;90(4):418–38.
22. Cecotti H. A self-paced and calibration-less SSVEP-based brain-computer interface speller. IEEE Trans Neural Syst Rehabil Eng. 2010;18(2):127–33.
23. Pfurtscheller G, Lopes da Silva FH. Event-related EEG/MEG synchronization and desynchronization: basic principles. Clin Neurophysiol. 1999;110(11):1842–57.
24. Pfurtscheller G, Neuper C, Flotzinger D, Pregenzer M. EEG-based discrimination between imagination of right and left hand movement. Electroencephalogr Clin Neurophysiol. 1997; 103(6):642–51.
25. Scherer R, Muller GR, Neuper C, et al. An asynchronously controlled EEG-based virtual keyboard: improvement of the spelling rate. IEEE Trans Biomed Eng. 2004;51(6):979–84.
26. Nijboer F, Furdea A, Gunst I, et al. An auditory brain-computer interface (BCI). J Neurosci Methods. 2008;167(1):43–50.
27. Birbaumer N. Slow cortical potentials: their origin, meaning, and clinical use. In: van Boxtel GJM, Bocker KBE, editors. Brain and behavior past, present, and future. Tilburg: Tilburg University Press; 1997. p. 25–39.
28. Elbert T, Rockstroh B, Lutzenberger W, Birbaumer N. Biofeedback of slow cortical potentials. I. Electroencephalogr Clin Neurophysiol. 1980;48(3):293–301.
29. Vidal JJ. Toward direct brain-computer communication. Annu Rev Biophys Bioeng. 1973;2:157–80.
30. Thut G, Nietzel A, Brandt SA, Pascual-Leone A. Alpha-band electroencephalographic activity over occipital cortex indexes visuospatial attention bias and predicts visual target detection. J Neurosci. 2006;26(37):9494–502.
31. Kelly SP, Lalor EC, Reilly RB, Foxe JJ. Increases in alpha oscillatory power reflect an active retinotopic mechanism for distracter suppression during sustained visuospatial attention. J Neurophysiol. 2006;95(6):3844–51.
32. van Gerven M, Jensen O. Attention modulations of posterior alpha as a control signal for two-dimensional brain-computer interfaces. J Neurosci Methods. 2009;179(1):78–84.
33. Kwong KK, Belliveau JW, Chesler DA, et al. Dynamic magnetic resonance imaging of human brain activity during primary sensory stimulation. Proc Natl Acad Sci USA. 1992;89(12):5675–9.
34. Boly M, Coleman MR, Davis MH, et al. When thoughts become action: an fMRI paradigm to study volitional brain activity in non-communicative brain injured patients. Neuroimage. 2007;36(3):979–92.
35. Monti M, Colemand MR, Owen AM. "Brain-reading" with real-time fMRI: communication via detection of brain states in the absence of motor response. In: 14th annual meeting of the organization for the human brain mapping. Melbourne: Elsevier; 2008. p. 133.
36. Irani F, Platek SM, Bunce S, et al. Functional near infrared spectroscopy (fNIRS): an emerging neuroimaging technology with important applications for the study of brain disorders. Clin Neuropsychol. 2007;21(1):9–37.

37. Coyle SM, Ward TE, Markham CM. Brain-computer interface using a simplified functional near-infrared spectroscopy system. J Neural Eng. 2007;4(3):219–26.
38. Luu S, Chau T. Decoding subjective preference from single-trial near-infrared spectroscopy signals. J Neural Eng. 2009;6(1):016003.
39. Sitaram R, Zhang H, Guan C, et al. Temporal classification of multichannel near-infrared spectroscopy signals of motor imagery for developing a brain-computer interface. Neuroimage. 2007;34(4):1416–27.
40. Nijboer F, Sellers EW, Mellinger J, et al. A P300-based brain-computer interface for people with amyotrophic lateral sclerosis. Clin Neurophysiol. 2008;119(8):1909–16.
41. Lulé D, Noirhomme Q, Kleih S, et al. Probing command following in patients with disorders of consciousness using a brain-computer interface. Clin Neurophysiol (Accepted).
42. Kubler A, Kotchoubey B, Hinterberger T, et al. The thought translation device: a neurophysiological approach to communication in total motor paralysis. Exp Brain Res. 1999;124(2): 223–32.
43. Neuper C, Muller GR, Kubler A, et al. Clinical application of an EEG-based brain-computer interface: a case study in a patient with severe motor impairment. Clin Neurophysiol. 2003; 114(3):399–409.
44. Perelmouter J, Kotchoubey B, Kübler A, et al. Language support program for thought translation devices. Automedica. 1999;18:67–84.
45. Pfurtscheller G, Muller-Putz GR, Schlogl A, et al. 15 years of BCI research at Graz University of Technology: current projects. IEEE Trans Neural Syst Rehabil Eng. 2006;14(2):205–10.
46. Cruse D, Bekinschtein TA, Monti M, Owen AM. Detecting awareness in the vegetative state with EEG. In: 16th annual meeting of the organization for human brain mapping. Barcelona: Elsevier; 2010.
47. Birbaumer N, Ghanayim N, Hinterberger T, et al. A spelling device for the paralysed. Nature. 1999;398(6725):297–8.
48. Birbaumer N, Kubler A, Ghanayim N, et al. The thought translation device (TTD) for completely paralyzed patients. IEEE Trans Rehabil Eng. 2000;8(2):190–3.
49. Monti MM, Vanhaudenhuyse A, Coleman MR, et al. Willful modulation of brain activity in disorders of consciousness. N Engl J Med. 2010;362:579–89.
50. Naito M, Michioka Y, Ozawa K, et al. A communication means for totally locked-in ALS patients based on changes in cerebral blood volume measured with near-infrared light. IEICE Trans Inf Syst. 2007;E90-D(7):1028–37.
51. Kennedy PR, Bakay RA. Restoration of neural output from a paralyzed patient by a direct brain connection. Neuroreport. 1998;9(8):1707–11.
52. Kennedy PR, Bakay RA, Moore MM, et al. Direct control of a computer from the human central nervous system. IEEE Trans Rehabil Eng. 2000;8(2):198–202.
53. Brumberg JS, Nieto-Castanon A, Kennedy PR, Guenther FH. Brain-computer interfaces for speech communication. Speech Commun. 2010;52(4):367–79.
54. Hinterberger T, Widman G, Lal TN, et al. Voluntary brain regulation and communication with electrocorticogram signals. Epilepsy Behav. 2008;13(2):300–6.
55. Leuthardt EC, Schalk G, Wolpaw JR, et al. A brain-computer interface using electrocorticographic signals in humans. J Neural Eng. 2004;1(2):63–71.
56. Hill NJ, Lal TN, Schroder M, et al. Classifying EEG and ECoG signals without subject training for fast BCI implementation: comparison of nonparalyzed and completely paralyzed subjects. IEEE Trans Neural Syst Rehabil Eng. 2006;14(2):183–6.
57. Blankertz B, Sannelli C, Halder S, et al. Neurophysiological predictor of SMR-based BCI performance. Neuroimage. 2010;51(4):1303–9.
58. Giacino J, Ashwal S, Childs N, et al. The minimally conscious state: definition and diagnostic criteria. Neurology. 2002;58(3):349–53.

Chapter 8
Using Transcranial Magnetic Stimulation to Measure Cerebral Connectivity in Patients with Disorders of Consciousness

Melanie Boly, Olivia Gosseries, Marie-Aurélie Bruno, Mario Rosanova, and Marcello Massimini

Assessment of the Level of Consciousness in Noncommunicative Brain Damaged Patients

The clinical assessment of patients with disorders of consciousness is based on repeated behavioral observations performed by trained clinicians. During the exam, spontaneous movements of the patient, or her/his responses to multisensory stimulations are studied and assessed according to specialized behavioral scales [1–4]. In this context, the clinician searches typically for (1) signs of consciousness of self or the environment; (2) sustainable, reproducible, or voluntary responses to tactile, auditory, or noxious stimuli; and (3) signs of language comprehension or expression [5]. If none of these behavioral characteristics can be detected during cautious and repeated examinations, the subject is considered unconscious [6], while patients showing nonreflexive behaviors but remaining unable to communicate are considered to be in minimally conscious state [7]. Thus, according to clinical definition of consciousness, the subjects are conscious if they can show they are. However, as motor functions are often impaired in severely brain damaged patients, it can also happen that a subject is conscious but unable to move or speak [8]. For this reason, while the detection of voluntary signs at the patient's bedside is considered sufficient to infer that the subject is conscious, their absence does not necessarily imply the absence of conscious perception [5, 9, 10].

M. Boly, M.D., Ph.D. (✉) • M.-A. Bruno, Ph.D. • O. Gosseries, M.Sc.
Coma Science Group, Research Cyclotron Center, University of Liège,
Allée du 6 Août, Sart Tilman B30, 4000 Liège, Belgium
e-mail: mboly@ulg.ac.be; ma.bruno@doct.ulg.ac.be; ogosseries@doct.ulg.ac.be

M. Rosanova, Ph.D. • M. Massimini, Ph.D.
Physiology Department, University of Milan,
Via G.B. Grassi, 74, 20157 Milan, Italy
e-mail: mario.rosanova@gmail.com; marcello.massimini@gmail.com

C. Schnakers, S. Laureys (eds.), *Coma and Disorders of Consciousness*,
DOI 10.1007/978-1-4471-2440-5_8, © Springer-Verlag London 2012

Recently, the development of new functional neuroimaging paradigms allowed detecting signs of consciousness in patients completely unable to move [9]. For example, in a recent study [11], a patient in clinical vegetative state, seemingly not conscious, was scanned with the instruction to imagine playing tennis or wandering around her home. Remarkably, the patient showed a functional MRI activation similar to that found in healthy volunteers while instructed to perform these tasks. This case demonstrates that this patient was able to follow commands using thoughts, even if a motor response was absent. However, there are many cases where a patient could not show positive response to this paradigm, and nevertheless, be conscious. For example, the presence of aphasia, akinetic mutism, catatonic depression, or diffuse dopaminergic lesions could compromise this type of response to command, despite the presence of cognition [9]. Moreover, because of frequent movement artifacts and of possible alterations of neurovascular coupling, the acquisition and interpretation of functional MRI data in patients with disorders of consciousness are particularly challenging [12].

For these reasons, the absence of voluntary cerebral activity in the functional MRI scanner, as the absence of clinical response to command, does not imply an absence of consciousness. The behavioral approach and the active functional imaging paradigms represent two levels where a communication can be established with patients with disorders of consciousness and where a diagnosis of preserved consciousness can be performed. However, in the case of a negative result, these two methods leave the question of the presence or absence of consciousness unanswered.

Using Transcranial Magnetic Stimulation and EEG to Assess the Brain's Capacity to Generate Consciousness

We recently proposed an additional level where consciousness can be studied even if the subject is unable to communicate, clinically or via neural activity [13]. This paradigm aims at directly assessing the ability of the subject's brain to generate conscious perception, by assessing some properties of cerebral activity, which are theoretically pertinent in this context. This possibility requires (1) starting from a theory that suggests which properties are fundamental in the organization of a system to generate conscious experience (2) identifying and implementing a measure which practically allows detecting these properties in the brain. Here, we will take the example of integrated information theory [14], which stipulates that consciousness is equivalent to integrated information and that a physical system should be capable of generating conscious perception to the extent that it can enter in a large number of different states (information), without being breakable into a collection of independent subsystems (integration). Then, a concrete method is set up, in order to evaluate the brain's ability to integrate information. To this aim, a combination of transcranial magnetic stimulation and EEG is used (TMS-EEG). This technique allows to directly stimulate different assemblies of cortical neurons and record the immediate response of the rest of the brain. This method has been suggested to be an efficient way to appreciate, in a general level, in which extent different regions of thalamocortical system can interact globally (integration) and produce specific responses (information). Though this approach does not aim at asserting if a subject is really conscious or not, it may represent an objective way to evaluate brain ability to generate conscious perception.

Validation Studies Using This Technique

Before being applied to patients, TMS-EEG technique requires some validation works in different altered states of consciousness, in order to check its predictive value for detecting the level of consciousness of the subjects. Promising studies were performed during sleep and anesthesia, testing the theoretical predictions underlying this technique. These studies showed that during these diminished consciousness states, brain responses indeed lose the characteristics commonly observed during wakefulness. The first study was performed during slow-wave sleep, a state where the conscious content of the subjects is known to be greatly reduced. In contrary to the rich connectivity observed during wakefulness, brain responses to TMS are typically local, and a loss of integration is observed [15] (Fig. 8.1). If a more widespread response is observed, it will be stereotypical, propagating homogeneously in the brain, and losing all the complexity observed during wakefulness [16].

A second study [17] was recently performed during deep sedation obtained using the pharmacological agent midazolam. This study confirmed that when subjects lose consciousness, the response to TMS is very different from that observed during wakefulness, with typically local and stereotypical response, mimicking a local slow wave, which does not propagate to the rest of the cortex. Brain connectivity is then dramatically reduced, particularly in long-distance connections, and the response does not persist more than a few tens of milliseconds – in contrast to the more complex and long lasting response observed during wakefulness. This result suggests that loss of consciousness during anesthesia may also be linked to a loss of brain integration. Moreover, the stereotypical aspect of the response suggests a loss of brain areas specialization, i.e., a loss of information [18].

During sleep as under anesthesia, the homogenous and stereotypical response observed after TMS administration is thought to be generated not only due to a loss of cerebral integration, but also to a disappearance of the specialization of the different brain areas (loss of information), due to the presence of bistable dynamics. Bistable dynamics are generated in a system when the neurons reach a certain threshold of hyperpolarization. In contrary to the rich diversity of responses that can be obtained during wakefulness, the occurrence of this type of dynamics will induce a stereotypical behavior, with only all or nonresponses following a perturbation of the system. This type of dynamics has been suggested to be particularly unfavorable to the generation of integrated information in the brain, and to the generation of conscious perception [14, 19, 20].

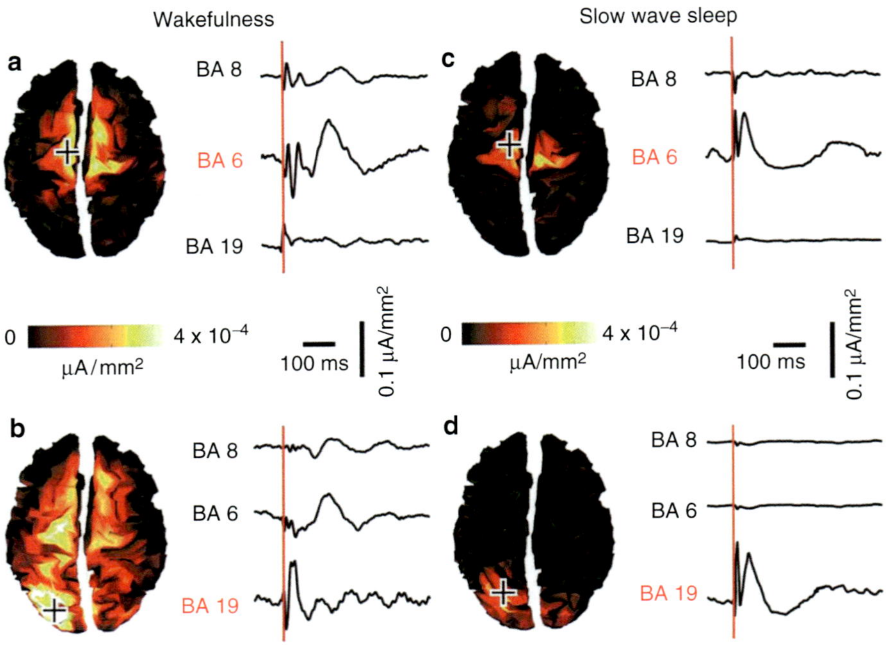

Fig. 8.1 Loss of integration and differentiation during slow-wave sleep. TMS is applied to frontal and occipital cortex during wakefulness (**a, b**) and slow-wave sleep (**c, d**). After source reconstruction, nonparametric statistics are applied in order to detect currents significantly evoked by the response to TMS. For each condition, significant currents recorded during the whole poststimulation period are displayed on cortical surface. On the right of each cortical surface, the temporal profiles of signals recorded in three brain areas (Brodmann areas 8, 6, and 19) are displayed (the stimulation time being shown as a *red* mark). During transition from wakefulness to slow-wave sleep, distant cortical areas cease to be influenced by the stimulation, suggesting a loss of brain integration. Moreover, brain responses to TMS become stereotypical, suggesting a loss of brain activity differentiation (Reproduced with permission from Massimini et al. [13])

Perspectives

The TMS-EEG could in principle be applied to brain damaged patients to evaluate their residual capacity to present a conscious experience. Beforehand, however, the acquisition of normative data should ideally be realized in order to define the normal or abnormal character of a given brain response, and to obtain quantitative measures related to these normality criteria. Some work has already been performed in this direction [21, 22], but it should be extended to a larger population and a larger number of brain areas in order to be more generally predictive. Second, a standardized analysis procedure should be set up in order to extract from TMS-EEG data some indexes, capturing in a synthetic manner the brain's ability to generate integrated information. For example, indexes using the entropy of the TMS-evoked response, or its algorithmic complexity could be useful tools in order to summarize the brain's ability to produce responses that are both integrated and specific (information). This type of measure would be low for a modular system, because in this case, the activity would remain local; it would also be low for networks with widespread but homogeneous connectivity, because all the elements would respond in the same way. In theory, only the networks that are both integrated and differentiated could react to TMS with a response presenting a high complexity. Before applying this technique for the diagnosis of brain damaged patients, other studies should be performed using other anesthetic agents (e.g., propofol, ketamine, xenon, sevoflurane) and different levels of sedation, in order to extend previously obtained results. Indeed, a reliable marker of consciousness level should behave in the same way in various altered states of consciousness, the etiology of which being physiological (sleep), pharmacological (anesthesia), or pathological (coma, vegetative state and related disorders). Even if the preliminary studies show very encouraging results, these findings, thus, should be validated on a larger number of subjects and conditions before the application of this technique for clinical diagnosis.

References

1. Giacino JT, Kalmar K, Whyte J. The JFK coma recovery scale-revised: measurement characteristics and diagnostic utility. Arch Phys Med Rehabil. 2004;85(12):2020–9.
2. Gill-Thwaites H, Munday R. The sensory modality assessment and rehabilitation technique (SMART): a valid and reliable assessment for vegetative state and minimally conscious state patients. Brain Inj. 2004;18(12):1255–69.
3. Kalmar K, Giacino JT. The JFK coma recovery scale–revised. Neuropsychol Rehabil. 2005;15(3–4):454–60.
4. Shiel A, Horn SA, Wilson BA, et al. The wessex head injury matrix (WHIM) main scale: a preliminary report on a scale to assess and monitor patient recovery after severe head injury. Clin Rehabil. 2000;14(4):408–16.
5. Laureys S, Owen AM, Schiff ND. Brain function in coma, vegetative state, and related disorders. Lancet Neurol. 2004;3(9):537–46.
6. The Multi-Society Task Force on PVS. Medical aspects of the persistent vegetative state (1). N Engl J Med. 1994;330(21):1499–508.
7. Giacino JT, Ashwal S, Childs N, et al. The minimally conscious state: definition and diagnostic criteria. Neurology. 2002;58(3):349–53.
8. Schnakers C, Perrin F, Schabus M, et al. Detecting consciousness in a total locked-in syndrome: an active event-related paradigm. Neurocase. 2009;15(4):271–7.
9. Boly M, Coleman MR, Davis MH, et al. When thoughts become action: an fMRI paradigm to study volitional brain activity in non-communicative brain injured patients. Neuroimage. 2007;36(3):979–92.
10. Monti MM, Vanhaudenhuyse A, Coleman MR, et al. Willful modulation of brain activity in disorders of consciousness. N Engl J Med. 2010;362(7):579–89.
11. Owen AM, Coleman MR, Boly M, et al. Detecting awareness in the vegetative state. Science. 2006;313(5792):1402.
12. Giacino JT, Hirsch J, Schiff N, Laureys S. Functional neuroimaging applications for assessment and rehabilitation planning in patients with disorders of consciousness. Arch Phys Med Rehabil. 2006;87(12):67–76.
13. Massimini M, Boly M, Casali A, et al. A perturbational approach for evaluating the brain's capacity for consciousness. Prog Brain Res. 2009;177:201–14.
14. Tononi G. Consciousness as integrated information: a provisional manifesto. Biol Bull. 2008;215(3):216–42.

15. Massimini M, Ferrarelli F, Huber R, et al. Breakdown of cortical effective connectivity during sleep. Science. 2005;309(5744):2228–32.
16. Massimini M, Ferrarelli F, Esser SK, et al. Triggering sleep slow waves by transcranial magnetic stimulation. Proc Natl Acad Sci USA. 2007;104(20):8496–501.
17. Ferrarelli F, Massimini M, Sarasso S, et al. Breakdown in cortical effective connectivity during midazolam-induced loss of consciousness. Proc Natl Acad Sci USA. 2010;107(6):2681–6.
18. Alkire MT, Hudetz AG, Tononi G. Consciousness and anesthesia. Science. 2008;322(5903): 876–80.
19. Tononi G, Massimini M. Why does consciousness fade in early sleep? Ann N Y Acad Sci. 2008;1129:330–4.
20. Boly M, Massimini M, Tononi G. Theoretical approaches to the diagnosis of altered states of consciousness. Prog Brain Res. 2009;177:383–98.
21. Casarotto S, Romero Lauro LJ, Bellina V, et al. EEG responses to TMS are sensitive to changes in the perturbation parameters and repeatable over time. PLoS One. 2010;5(4):10281.
22. Rosanova M, Casali A, Bellina V, et al. Natural frequencies of human corticothalamic circuits. J Neurosci. 2009;29(24):7679–85.

Chapter 9
Sleep in Disorders of Consciousness

Victor Cologan and Manuel Schabus

Introduction

Today consciousness is considered as multifaceted concept having two major components: arousal and awareness. Arousal refers to the level of consciousness (i.e., vigilance) and is supported by brainstem neuronal populations projecting to both thalamic and cortical areas. Awareness refers to the content of consciousness (i.e., awareness of the self and of the environment) and relies on the functional integrity of the cerebral cortex and its subcortical connections. Both components progressively decrease as sleep deepens. In some pathological situations, however, arousal and awareness are dissociated. This, for instance, is the case of patients in coma, vegetative state (VS) (today preferentially referred to as unresponsive wakefulness syndrome, UWS), or minimally conscious state (MCS). The question thus arises whether and in which ways sleep in severely brain-injured patients is being altered. It has been proposed that besides "offline" neuronal plasticity, one of the major functions of sleep is to restore general homeostasis (including, more specifically, subcortical brain structures) and to stabilize neuronal connections. Accordingly, alterations in sleep in DOC (Disorders of Consciousness) might be associated to a lower probability of recovery.

V. Cologan, M.Sc.
Coma Science Group, Cyclotron Research Center, University of Liège,
Allée du 6 Août, Sart Tilman B30, 4000 Liège, Belgium
e-mail: vcologan@student.ulg.ac.be

M. Schabus, Ph.D. (✉)
Coma Science Group, Cyclotron Research Center, University of Liège,
Allée du 6 Août, Sart Tilman B30, 4000 Liège, Belgium

Laboratory for Sleep and Consciousness Research, Department of Psychology,
University of Salzburg, Hellbrunnerstr. 34, Salzburg 5020 Austria
e-mail: manuel.schabus@sbg.ac.at

C. Schnakers, S. Laureys (eds.), *Coma and Disorders of Consciousness*,
DOI 10.1007/978-1-4471-2440-5_9, © Springer-Verlag London 2012

Polysomnography (PSG), which is the only valid sleep recording method, can be used to perform a clinical assessment of that kind. In particular, it provides useful information for the characterization of altered brain activity and prognosis. Most of the present research has been conducted on the acute phase of coma (i.e., immediately following brain injury) or on patients having already recovered consciousness. Little is known about the transitional states leading to recovery (VS/UWS, MCS) and other clinical entities such as locked-in syndrome (LIS) or brain death.

Sleep abnormalities are common in critically ill patients. In brain-injured patients, about half of the total sleep time occurs during the daytime and the circadian rhythm is often significantly diminished or even lost. Generally, these patients exhibit more frequent arousals and awakenings than healthy volunteers, and decreases in rapid eye movement (REM) sleep and deep non-REM sleep are common. Additionally to brain injury, considerable sleep disruption also arises from hospital environments throughout day and night. This is worth mentioning as sleep deprivation is known to have major and devastating impacts on mood, daytime fatigue, residual cognitive functioning, and the immune system, especially critical for brain-injured patients.

Studying Sleep in DOC

Although it is well-known that sleep abnormalities are common in critically ill patients, their mechanisms remain poorly understood and their fine-grained characterizations are still unknown [1]. First of all, one has to characterize the differences found in DOC patients as compared to those in healthy individuals. From a behavioral point of view, normal sleep is usually preceded by the search for a safe place, a progressive but reversible decrease of responsiveness to external stimuli and a decrease of motor output. In DOC, assessing these behavioral criteria is challenging and rarely conclusive. From a physiological point of view, normal sleep is associated with well-described cycles, stages, arousals, and microstructures (e.g., K-complexes, spindles). Yet the traditional scoring manual from Rechtschaffen and Kales [2] is often not appropriate for clinical contexts as summarized elsewhere [3]. In DOC, the classification of sleep and the existence of polysomnographic elements (of "unusual" shape or frequency characteristic), therefore, remains a matter of scientific debate.

Together with evidence of eye opening, the presence of a sleep–wake cycle defines the threshold for the progression from a comatose state to VS/UWS or MCS. However, despite the importance of a sleep–wake cycle for differential diagnosis, there is little empirical evidence that DOC patients actually exhibit classical sleep phenomena or display a circadian rhythm. Sleep–wake cycles are typically indirectly inferred by behavioral observations with prolonged periods of opened or closed eyes. Yet, as circadian rhythms are endogenously generated by a biological "Zeitgeber" located in the hypothalamic suprachiasmatic nucleus (SCN), it would be needed that more direct measures, such as the SCN controlled pineal hormone melatonin, are adopted. Note that a handful of studies conducted in intensive care units indicate the loss of circadian secretion of melatonin in sedated unresponsive patients [4].

Past studies reported day–night brain state differences in some but not other VS patients using continuous EEG [5]. Furthermore, it was shown that heart rate and blood pressure do not show the typical nocturnal decrease during night hours in traumatic VS [6]. However, an inherent problem to studies of that kind is daytime sleep, which decreases the amount of sleep during the nightly recording times. Another study in persistent VS patients showed significant circadian changes in body temperature and urinary excretion of hormones and sodium but revealed no changes in blood pressure or pulse rate [7]. In a more recent study by Bekinschtein and colleagues [8] it was reported that while VS/UWS patients with traumatic brain injury exhibit well-formed circadian temperature rhythms, patients with anoxic-hypoxic origin demonstrate no cycles or rhythmic behavior.

These findings suggest that the preservation of circadian rhythm may not only vary with the patients' state of consciousness, but also the extent of their individual brain damage.

It appears that the existence of sleep and its characterization in DOC is a most challenging issue as these patients do not show the normal behavioral, physiological, and regulatory signs of sleep. Circadian and homeostatic factors are potent modulators of sleep and it is, therefore, surprising that previous studies did not investigate in greater detail their existence and possible diagnostic and prognostic value before focusing on macro- or microstructural sleep changes. To this end, the detection of changes in hormonal plasma levels (e.g., melatonin, cortisol), temperature, along with those of blood pressure, heart rate, and actimetry monitoring should be performed first to accurately outline circadian variations in DOC.

The remaining question is the assessment of residual homeostasis in DOC. Unlike sleep patterns, homeostasis is rarely addressed in DOC. Support for the presence of homeostatic sleep regulation in DOC could be provided by simple wake extension protocols and by comparing the EEG before and after a period during which patients are prevented from sleep, e.g., behaviorally by stimulating externally during prolonged eye closure. A recent study by Landsness and colleagues [9] demonstrated, besides regular alternating NREM/REM sleep patterns, a clear homeostatic decline of EEG slow-wave activity across the night in all tested MCS but not VS/UWS patients. The study of homeostatic regulation of slow-wave activity might, therefore, provide a complementary tool of brain function for the near future.

Finally, previous studies on coma suggested that the presence of certain EEG patterns may be reliable markers for favorable outcome [10, 11]. It was reported that sleep patterns continue to become more "complex" (i.e., NREM–REM alterations, reappearance of sleep spindles, etc.) during rehabilitation therapy, sometimes even in parallel to patients' cognitive recovery [12]. Some authors have used Rechtschaffen and Kales sleep criteria to analyze the polysomnographic data in DOC [11, 13]. However, as many forms of brain damage may result in a relatively similar clinical state of unconsciousness and as modification of brain activity in DOC may substantially differ from physiological sleep patterns described by Rechtschaffen and Kales, those criteria are hardly applicable for scoring sleep in severely brain damaged patients. These scoring criteria do need update and revision in order to become fully suitable for sleep–wake assessment in DOC.

In conclusion, the study of sleep is of particular interest in DOC with various different etiologies as it might allow to identify relationships between specific PSG graphoelements and underlying functional neuroanatomy. Specifically, NREM sleep spindles and slow-wave sleep may reflect the preserved functional integrity of the thalamocortical network; present REM sleep may reflect residual functioning of brainstem nuclei including pons and adjacent portions of the midbrain; and last but not least the integrity of circadian organization of sleep–wake patterns might be informative of residual hypothalamic and suprachiasmatic nucleus (SCN) functioning.

Methodological Issues

In intensive care units, environmental factors are often not optimal for good sleep [1]. For example, not perfectly adjusted mechanical ventilation may cause significant sleep disruption. Further factors contributing to sleep abnormalities in intensive care units include acute pain, discomfort, increased alertness induced by continuous exposure to light or noise, as well as nutrition and nursing activities. In this context, important to note is the fact that sleep deprivation is known to have negative impact on immune and endocrine functions. It also induces sympathetic activation and elevation of blood pressure, which in turn can increase morbidity. It is, therefore, suggested that in order to support optimal recovery and promote good neurobehavioral functioning, clinicians should be aware of these basic facts.

PSG is the only tool allowing reliable evaluation of sleep. Yet, recording good quality signals in DOC is very challenging due to artifacts caused by strong perspiration, thermal dysregulation, skin and skull lesions, or electrical artifacts from life-supporting devices. When looking at the basic EEG structure, the first examination to make is to test for reactivity, i.e., to check for a change in EEG caused by external sensory stimulation. Painful or auditory stimuli are usually used for this purpose and the presence of EEG reactivity often indicates a less severe disorder [14]. Another evaluation, although rarely used in comatose patients, concerns arousal organization during sleep. Arousals can be defined as simultaneous changes of EEG along with autonomic system or somatic activity [15]. Compared to healthy individuals, DOC patients do not exhibit normal arousal alternations or cyclic alternating patterns (CAPs) [16]. In these patients, changes in brain activation may be considerably slowed, lasting a number of seconds or even minutes, and are often not rhythmic. Arousal alternations are often more extreme than normal and may even become life-threatening, especially those occurring in the vegetative system (e.g., involving cerebrospinal fluid pressure increase) [17]. These extreme sleep microstructure changes seen in DOC indicate that arousal control mechanisms have been injured or severely altered.

The advantage of EEG recordings over functional neuroimaging includes its high temporal resolution and its noninvasive nature, along with its portability and low cost. Its main limitation is the spatial resolution and current lack of specificity (diffuse slowing of background rhythms is, e.g., seen in various encephalopathies regardless of the etiology). High-density EEG is one current development that will allow better spatial source reconstruction, yet the spatial resolution of functional magnetic resonance imaging (fMRI) including the assessment of deep brain structures remains unattainable. It is also to be noted that EEG is often heavily contaminated by uncontrolled eye movements and muscle activation occurring in DOC. Sophisticated correction methods, e.g., various independent component analysis (ICA) algorithms, may be necessary in order to obtain clean EEG data exploitable for in-depth analysis and scientific as well as clinical interpretation.

Coma

Prevalent alpha or (alpha-coma, AC), spindle-like activity (spindle-coma, SC), and triphasic waves are the most typical EEG patterns observed in coma patients [14]. In AC, alpha activity between 8 and 12 Hz dominates the frequency spectrum and presents an usual widespread topography with often high amplitude at frontal electrodes and no reactivity to eye opening as usually observed (i.e., no posterior block of alpha oscillations). Alpha coma patterns have been described after hypoxia as well as drug intoxications. SC is a chronic electrophysiological pattern in which physiological sleep components, specifically sleep spindles (9–14 Hz) are superimposed on a background of delta (0.9–4 Hz) and theta (4–8 Hz) activity. Triphasic waves consist in bursts of moderate to high amplitude (100–300 μV) activity, usually of 1.5–2.5 Hz, and frequently predominating in frontal regions. The initial negative component is the sharpest, whereas the following positive portion of the complex is the largest and is followed by another negative wave. Triphasic waves are usually bisynchronous but may show shifting asymmetries. Persistent asymmetry suggests an underlying structural lesion on the side of the lower amplitude.

In humans, the pathophysiological mechanism of SC has been related to the pontine raphe nuclei and thalamocortical circuits together with the impairment of the ascending reticular activating system located in the midbrain, which usually maintains arousal [18–20]. SC is considered to be a more "benign" condition than AC, and is largely related to lower cerebral damages. Indeed, the overall mortality in case of SC does not exceed 25% [21]. This quite good prognosis might be explained by the preservation of thalamocortical functioning, which underlies spindle generation [22].

Generally, EEG sleep patterns have been considered as favorable prognostic markers in brain-injured patients [10, 11] and it has been shown that sleep patterns continue to normalize during rehabilitation together with the recovery of cognitive functioning [12]. The presence of organized sleep patterns is also predictive of good outcome [23, 24]. In contrast, patients showing only monophasic EEG (i.e., continuous low voltage theta-delta activity) or CAPs indicating arousal

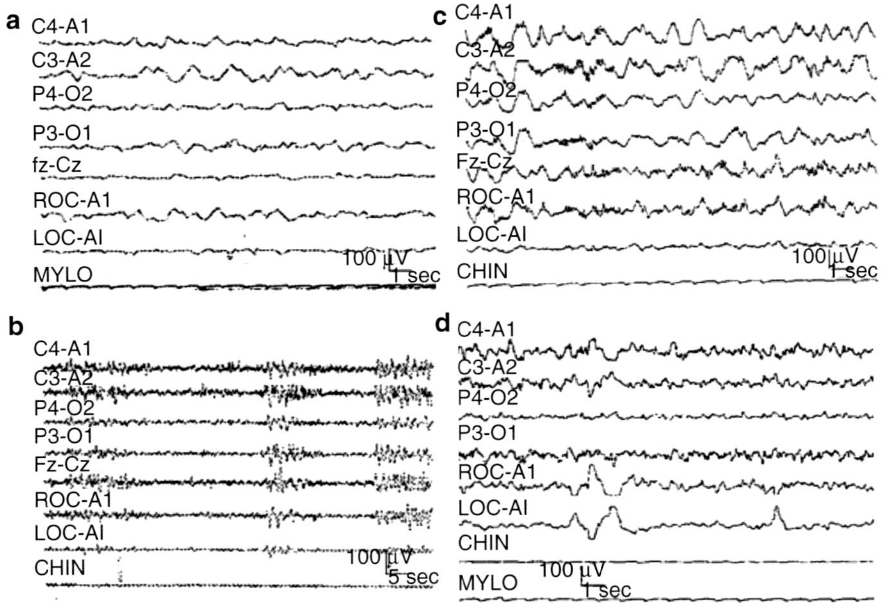

Fig. 9.1 Polysomnographic recordings in subacute (7–14 days post onset) comatose patients. (**a**) Panels depict a monophasic EEG with continuous low voltage theta-delta activity as well as (**b**) recurrent abnormal (CAP) activity both indicative of bad outcome. The recovery of (**c**) NREM sleep with well-structure spindles as well as the reappearance of REM sleep (**d**), on the other hand, has been related to good outcome (Adapted from [24])

instability during NREM sleep, in the absence of classical sleep elements, have been associated with bad outcome (death or severe disabilities). Especially REM sleep elements (rapid ocular movements, muscle twitches, saw-tooth waves), alternating regularly with NREM sleep elements as well as certain NREM sleep elements such as K-complexes and sleep spindles themselves, have been related to good outcome (full recovery or only mild disability). Figure 9.1 illustrates some of the key patterns discussed above (modified from [24]).

The reappearance of regular sleep patterns and specifically sleep spindles is of good prognosis in comatose patients. While the absence of spindles in coma presumably results from the interruption of either the ascending reticulothalamocortical pathway or thalamocortical loops, the absence of sleep–wake cycles, which is also typical in comatose patients, is associated with brainstem dysfunction.

These sleep patterns are associated to functional outcome as they allow a glimpse into the residual connectivity of the lesioned brain. For example, it has been suggested that the amount or intensity of sleep spindles reflects intact and efficiently connected thalamocortical networks, as supported by recent data associating high general cognitive and memory abilities to high spindle activity during the night [25, 26]. In conclusion, the magnitude of observed sleep alterations seems to be related to injury severity.

"Vegetative State" / "Unresponsive Wakefulness Syndrome"

Patients in VS (today increasingly termed UWS) are unresponsive to external stimuli and are usually considered to be unconscious and unaware. Patients in this state have a total loss of forebrain function but preservation of brainstem functions including breathing, swallowing, or cranial nerve reflexes. Occasionally, VS patients exhibit electrocerebral inactivity (i.e., no cerebral activity over 2 μV), although the majority show some EEG activity. Unlike comatose patients, VS patients open and close their eyes and thereby exhibit–at least at a behavioral level–behavior that resembles normal sleep–wake cycling.

Patients in the full VS (formerly called *apallic syndrome*) often show severe sleep fragmentation, which is likely caused by structural changes in brain areas responsible for sleep maintenance, as well as absent sleep spindling [27, 28]. However, patients close to remission often show reappearance of NREM and REM sleep stages, together with an increase in total sleep time, as well as sleep spindle activity [29]. With regards to REM sleep, these patients exhibit significantly less phasic REM events such as rapid eye movements, chin and leg muscle twitches [13]. Yet, preserved sleep-related erections similar to those in normal subjects [30] and nystagmus (which is an involuntary and jerky oscillatory movement of the eyes different from that observed in REM sleep) [31] are reported in the literature.

It is discussed that this reduction of phasic rapid eye movements and muscles twitches during REM sleep may reflect damage to the cholinergic mechanisms of the pedunculopontine tegmentum (PPT).

Recovered State

It appears that also brain-injured patients who recover consciousness (exit-MCS or recovered state) still suffer from various sleep disturbances. Insomnia-like sleep complaints (i.e., sleeplessness) are reported as much as hypersomnia-like complaints (i.e., excessive amount of sleepiness) and are probably physiologically linked to structural changes in brain arousal systems [32–36]. Frequently, as seen in normal insomnia patients, DOC patients do overestimate the degree of their sleep disturbance as revealed when comparing subjective (sleep diaries) and objective (actigraphy, polysomnography) sleep data [37]. Beside these alterations, sleep pattern and sleep onset latency modifications are common, with deep NREM sleep being most preserved [38–41].

Fatigue, mood disturbances, and exacerbated cognitive deficits as well as weakening of immune function are among the consequences of chronic sleep alterations in brain injured patients. Treatment attempts in this population appear rather scarce. Although for short-term treatment of sleep disorders the prescription of hypnotic medications may be an effective approach, long-term use of these medications is problematic, probably even more so than in non-brain-injured individuals. Nonpharmacological treatments like psychotherapeutic intervention [42] or instrumental conditioning of specific brain oscillations (neurofeedback) [43] may offer an alternative, yet longer than normal intervention durations have to be expected.

Locked-in Syndrome

The literature about sleep in LIS patients is especially scarce. Brain lesions in these patients affect the ventropontine area sparing the pontine tegmentum. A concomitant cerebellum lesion is frequent as there is a rupture of the basilar artery. The observed spectrum of altered sleep in LIS can vary from almost normal sleep patterns [44] to hyposomnia [45], disorganized NREM sleep [46–50], or complete REM absence [46, 47, 50, 51]. This wide spectrum is most likely explained by differences in the exact location and extent of causative lesions. Thus, LIS patients can present in rare cases no major sleep abnormalities although severe neurological deficits are evident. Specifically, it appears that the more extended the pontine lesion, the more pronounced the sleep disturbance, especially affecting REM sleep. Lesion severity increases in case of bilateral or dorsal extensions, and of pontine tegmentum involvement, especially if the serotonin-releasing raphe nuclei of the brainstem (medial portion of the reticular formation) are included.

As mentioned previously, careful attention must be given to the environmental factors (light, noise, nightly nursing activities) in which sleep disorders emerge in these patients. This is specifically important for LIS patients who are completely aware of their environment and who likewise suffer from the consequences of inadequate sleep, yet they are (paralyzed and mute) "locked-in" their bodies.

Conclusion

In summary, DOCs are often linked to alterations in sleep architecture and its microstructure. In the comatose state, the patient by definition shows no eye-opening and no sleep–wake cycling. However, certain NREM and REM graphoelements may emerge, yet in an often unusual generalized form. In the VS/UWS, patients by definition show transient periods of eye-opening and sleep–wake cycles. However, very few studies provide empirical evidence of the residual sleep architecture. Most literature exists for the recovery from coma and deals with the reappearance of NREM graphoelements such as sleep spindles. In these patients hypersomnia and insomnia appear to be common phenomena, which ask to be appropriately addressed and treated in the future. It has to be noted that older studies might have mixed the two clinical entities VS and MCS as the latter entity was only defined in 2002 by Giacino.

In the LIS (as a special case outside the classical DOC spectrum), sleep alterations are very variable and depend mainly on the extent and location of the brainstem lesion.

To date there are no clearly defined polysomnographic patterns that reliably define each of the reviewed DOC states. In addition, there is very little evidence indicating whether sleep in DOC is still under normal circadian and homeostatic control. Future studies should, therefore, aim for long-term PSG recordings together with circadian measures in well-documented patients. These tools might in the long run help to further differentiate the various DOC states, and especially complement the often difficult distinction between VS/UWS and MCS patients (for review also see [52]). In addition, certain sleep patterns such as spindles seem predictive of later outcome, yet longitudinal sleep studies are still needed in order to come up with reliable outcome markers relevant for individual patients.

From a methodological point of view, it is true that studying sleep in DOC is a challenging endeavor. Long-term PSG of DOC patients in clinical or rehabilitation centers is difficult because of various artifacts arising from environmental and nursing activities or from clinical instability or mandatory medication conditions. Another major problem is that PSG signals in DOC are often so much altered that standard sleep criteria can hardly be used for sleep scoring.

The characterization of sleep and its relationships with arousal, homeostasis, and circadian rhythmicity is essential in order to further understand DOC conditions and might offer access to highly needed complementary diagnostic and prognostic information in this specific patient population.

References

1. Parthasarathy S, Tobin MJ. Sleep in the intensive care unit. Intensive Care Med. 2004; 30(2):197–206.
2. Rechtschaffen A, Kales A. A manual of standardized terminology, techniques and scoring system for sleep stages of human subjects. Bethesda: U.S. Department of Health, Education, and Welfare; 1968. p. 12.
3. Himanen SL, Hasan J. Limitations of Rechtschaffen and Kales. Sleep Med Rev. 2000;4(2): 149–67.
4. Mundigler G, et al. Impaired circadian rhythm of melatonin secretion in sedated critically ill patients with severe sepsis. Crit Care Med. 2002;30(3):536–40.
5. Isono M, et al. Sleep cycle in patients in a state of permanent unconsciousness. Brain Inj. 2002;16(8):705–12.
6. Pattoneri P, et al. Circadian blood pressure and heart rate changes in patients in a persistent vegetative state after traumatic brain injury. J Clin Hypertens (Greenwich). 2005;7(12):734–9.
7. Fukudome Y, et al. Circadian blood pressure in patients in a persistent vegetative state. Am J Physiol. 1996;270(5 Pt 2):R1109–14.
8. Bekinschtein TA, et al. Circadian rhythms in the vegetative state. Brain Inj. 2009;23(11): 915–9.
9. Landsness E, et al. Electrophysiological correlates of behavioural changes in vigilance in vegetative state and minimally conscious state. Brain. 2011;134(8):2222–32.
10. Bergamasco B, et al. The sleep cycle in coma: prognostic value. Electroencephalogr Clin Neurophysiol. 1968;25(1):87.
11. Chatrian GE, White Jr LE, Daly D. Electroencephalographic patterns resembling those of sleep in certain comatose states after injuries to the head. Electroencephalogr Clin Neurophysiol. 1963;15:272–80.

12. Ron S, et al. Time-related changes in the distribution of sleep stages in brain injured patients. Electroencephalogr Clin Neurophysiol. 1980;48(4):432–41.
13. Oksenberg A, et al. Phasic activities of rapid eye movement sleep in vegetative state patients. Sleep. 2001;24(6):703–6.
14. Brenner RP. The interpretation of the EEG in stupor and coma. Neurologist. 2005;11(5): 271–84.
15. Halasz P, et al. The nature of arousal in sleep. J Sleep Res. 2004;13(1):1–23.
16. Freedman NS, et al. Abnormal sleep/wake cycles and the effect of environmental noise on sleep disruption in the intensive care unit. Am J Respir Crit Care Med. 2001;163(2):451–7.
17. Evans BM. What does brain damage tell us about the mechanisms of sleep? J R Soc Med. 2002;95(12):591–7.
18. Britt Jr CW, Raso E, Gerson LP. Spindle coma, secondary to primary traumatic midbrain hemorrhage. Electroencephalogr Clin Neurophysiol. 1980;49(3–4):406–8.
19. Britt Jr CW. Nontraumatic "spindle coma": clinical, EEG, and prognostic features. Neurology. 1981;31(4):393–7.
20. Seet RC, Lim EC, Wilder-Smith EP. Spindle coma from acute midbrain infarction. Neurology. 2005;64(12):2159–60.
21. Kaplan PW, et al. Clinical correlates and prognosis in early spindle coma. Clin Neurophysiol. 2000;111(4):584–90.
22. Schabus M, et al. Hemodynamic cerebral correlates of sleep spindles during human non- REM sleep. Proc Natl Acad Sci USA. 2007;104(32):13164–9.
23. Evans BM, Bartlett JR. Prediction of outcome in severe head injury based on recognition of sleep related activity in the polygraphic electroencephalogram. J Neurol Neurosurg Psychiatry. 1995;59(1):17–25.
24. Valente M, et al. Sleep organization pattern as a prognostic marker at the subacute stage of post-traumatic coma. Clin Neurophysiol. 2002;113(11):1798–805.
25. Schabus M, et al. Sleep spindle-related activity in the human EEG and its relation to general cognitive and learning abilities. Eur J Neurosci. 2006;23(7):1738–46.
26. Bodizs R, et al. Prediction of general mental ability based on neural oscillation measures of sleep. J Sleep Res. 2005;14(3):285–92.
27. Giubilei F, et al. Sleep abnormalities in traumatic apallic syndrome. J Neurol Neurosurg Psychiatry. 1995;58(4):484–6.
28. D'Aleo G, et al. Sleep spindles in the initial stages of the vegetative state. Ital J Neurol Sci. 1994;15(7):347–51.
29. D'Aleo G, et al. Sleep in the last remission stages of vegetative state of traumatic nature. Funct Neurol. 1994;9(4):189–92.
30. Oksenberg A, et al. Sleep-related erections in vegetative state patients. Sleep. 2000;23(7): 953–7.
31. Gordon CR, Oksenberg A. Spontaneous nystagmus across the sleep-wake cycle in vegetative state patients. Electroencephalogr Clin Neurophysiol. 1993;86(2):132–7.
32. George B, Landau-Ferey J. Twelve months' follow-up by night sleep EEG after recovery from severe head trauma. Neurochirurgia (Stuttg). 1986;29(2):45–7.
33. Keshavan MS, Channabasavanna SM, Reddy GN. Post-traumatic psychiatric disturbances: patterns and predictors of outcome. Br J Psychiatry. 1981;138:157–60.
34. Cohen M, et al. Temporally related changes of sleep complaints in traumatic brain injured patients. J Neurol Neurosurg Psychiatry. 1992;55(4):313–5.
35. Clinchot DM, et al. Defining sleep disturbance after brain injury. Am J Phys Med Rehabil. 1998;77(4):291–5.
36. Fichtenberg NL, et al. Insomnia in a post-acute brain injury sample. Brain Inj. 2002;16(3): 197–206.
37. Ouellet MC, Savard J, Morin CM. Insomnia following traumatic brain injury: a review. Neurorehabil Neural Repair. 2004;18(4):187–98.
38. Guilleminault C, et al. Hypersomnia after head-neck trauma: a medicolegal dilemma. Neurology. 2000;54(3):653–9.

39. Masel BE, et al. Excessive daytime sleepiness in adults with brain injuries. Arch Phys Med Rehabil. 2001;82(11):1526–32.
40. Ouellet MC, Beaulieu-Bonneau S, Morin CM. Insomnia in patients with traumatic brain injury: frequency, characteristics, and risk factors. J Head Trauma Rehabil. 2006;21(3): 199–212.
41. Ouellet MC, Morin CM. Subjective and objective measures of insomnia in the context of traumatic brain injury: a preliminary study. Sleep Med. 2006;7(6):486–97.
42. Ouellet MC, Morin CM. Cognitive behavioral therapy for insomnia associated with traumatic brain injury: a single-case study. Arch Phys Med Rehabil. 2004;85(8):1298–302.
43. Hoedlmoser K, et al. Non-pharmacological alternatives for the treatment of insomnia—instrumental EEG conditioning, a new alternative? In: Soriento YE, editor. Melatonin, sleep and insomnia. New York: Nova; 2011. p. 69–101.
44. Oksenberg A, et al. Polysomnography in locked-in syndrome. Electroencephalogr Clin Neurophysiol. 1991;78(4):314–7.
45. Guilleminault C, Cathala JP, Castaigne P. Effects of 5-hydroxytryptophan on sleep of a patient with a brain-stem lesion. Electroencephalogr Clin Neurophysiol. 1973;34(2):177–84.
46. Markand ON, Dyken ML. Sleep abnormalities in patients with brain stem lesions. Neurology. 1976;26(8):769–76.
47. Cummings JL, Greenberg R. Sleep patterns in the "locked-in" syndrome. Electroencephalogr Clin Neurophysiol. 1977;43(2):270–1.
48. Freemon FR, Salinas-Garcia RF, Ward JW. Sleep patterns in a patient with a brain stem infarction involving the raphe nucleus. Electroencephalogr Clin Neurophysiol. 1974;36(6):657–60.
49. Autret A, et al. A syndrome of REM and non-REM sleep reduction and lateral gaze paresis after medial tegmental pontine stroke. Computed tomographic scans and anatomical correlations in four patients. Arch Neurol. 1988;45(11):1236–42.
50. Tamura K, et al. Disturbances of the sleep-waking cycle in patients with vascular brain stem lesions. Clin Electroencephalogr. 1983;14(1):35–46.
51. Lavie P, et al. Localized pontine lesion: nearly total absence of REM sleep. Neurology. 1984;34(1):118–20.
52. Cologan V, et al. Sleep in disorders of consciousness. Sleep Med Rev. 2010;14:97–105.

Chapter 10
Sensory Stimulation Program

Haibo Di and Caroline Schnakers

Introduction

Progress in intensive care has led to an increase in the number of patients who survive a severe brain lesion. Although the main part recovers in the first days following the coma, some of these patients stay in a disorder of consciousness. The medical care provided to these patients in neurology and neurorehabilitation units is usually mainly palliative and minimizes complications rather than improving the patients' recovery. Until now, few treatments were validated in patients with disorders of consciousness. Sensory stimulation programs constitute the treatment most frequently applied during the recovery of these patients. These programs are based on the principles of brain plasticity and of sensory deprivation [1].

The idea according to which an injured brain has the capacity to reorganize itself to compensate for the affected regions is broadly accepted for several years [2]. The most famous case illustrating this phenomenon is the case of Terry Wallis. Indeed, this patient remained for 19 years in a minimally conscious state after a traumatic brain injury. His spectacular recovery may be explained by this principle of brain plasticity. A study of Voss et al. revealed a neural change (mainly involving the cuneus and the precuneus) in this patient having recovered a functional verbal communication and motor activity [3]. These results stress the importance to develop therapeutics to optimize the brain plasticity and, hence, the full consciousness

H. Di, Ph.D. (✉)
Physiology Department, International Vegetative State and Consciousness Science Institute, Hangzhou Normal University, Xuelin, 310036 Hangzhou, Zhejiang, China
e-mail: dihaibo@yahoo.com.cn

C. Schnakers, Ph.D.
Coma Science Group, Cyclotron Research Center, University of Liège, Allée du 6 Août, Sart Tilman B30, 4000 Liège, Belgium
e-mail: c.schnakers@ulg.ac.be

C. Schnakers, S. Laureys (eds.), *Coma and Disorders of Consciousness*, DOI 10.1007/978-1-4471-2440-5_10, © Springer-Verlag London 2012

recovery in severely brain-injured adults. Providing sensory stimulations (auditory, verbal, visual, olfactory, tactile, and gustatory) to the patient could potentially stimulate affected neural networks, accelerate the brain plasticity, and avoid a sensory deprivation which could slow down the patient's consciousness recovery [1]. In this chapter, we will introduce the theoretical principles underlying these programs and the studies assessing their clinical interest. We will also discuss the limitations of this treatment and consider future directions for clinical research.

Theoretical Principles Related to Sensory Stimulation Programs

Sensory stimulation programs usually consist in presenting different types of environmental stimuli to the patient in order to optimize the consciousness level. These programs tend to avoid a sensory deprivation and to improve behavioral responses [4]. According to Ansell and Keenan [5], these programs allow the patients to follow a structured stimulation, optimizing their aptitude to react and to respond to their environment. These would constitute enriched environments that would potentially have an impact on the structure and the functions of the brain and, hence, on the brain plasticity.

Brain Plasticity

Years ago, neurologists considered that, after a brain lesion, neurons cannot recover anymore and the brain cannot become richer of new neurons. However, more recently, an increasing number of studies have revealed the remarkable capacity of young as well as old brain to adapt and transform itself according to the environment, to restructure connections between neurons in order to develop networks, which optimize the circulation of information provided by the environment. The adult nervous system would be malleable and, hence, sensitive to modifications and adaptations [6, 7].

Effects of an Enriched Environment on the Behavior, the Structure, and the Functions of the Brain

Sensory stimulation programs can be considered as enriched environments. The principle of "enriched environment" was used by researchers studying animal behavior. These experiments consisted in using ample animal boxes containing various objects stimulating curiosity and manipulation. It is one of the oldest approaches used to show that experiences can change the brain on a neuroanatomical and biochemical level [8, 9]. On a behavioral level, studies on animals allowed showing memory improvements in enriched environment in the course of adult life and during aging. At a neurobiological level, studies revealed that this environment leads to an increase in the thickness of the cortex and to cell modifications. Several studies performed in rats showed that their stay in enriched environments increases their capacity of learning, memory as well as their capacity of adaptation in comparison to rats staying in impoverished environments [10, 11]. Sensory stimulations would allow changes in the structure and the functioning of the nervous system but also in the behaviors that the individual can demonstrate to interact with his surroundings.

Previous Studies on Sensory Stimulation Programs

Considering these principles, the Institutes for the Achievement of Human Potential (IAHP) have introduced sensory stimulation programs in the neurorehabilitation field and, despite the lack of scientific evidence, have supported the idea, according to which these programs could enhance the synaptic reinnervation and, therefore, the recovery from coma in severely brain-injured patients [12].

Numerous studies investigated the interest of these sensory stimulations in patients with disorders of consciousness. The most part seems to show a positive effect of these programs on consciousness recovery [4, 12–21]. These results are, however, often affected by methodological biases and must be considered with caution. Indeed, Lombardi et al. assessed the efficacy of sensory stimulation programs in patients diagnosed as being in a coma or in a vegetative state [22] in performing a systematic review of randomized and nonrandomized controlled trials published from 1966 to 2002. This meta-analysis reported only three studies corresponding to the authors' criteria, the other ones being, for the most part, noncontrolled studies or descriptive case reports.

In the first study, Mitchell (1990) divided 24 severely brain-injured patients in two groups of 12 patients hospitalized in the same neurological unit (the control group and the experimental group) [17]. The control group was matched to the experimental group according to the age, the gender, the brain lesion, and the Glasgow Coma Scale (GCS) score at the admission. The experimental treatment involved visual, auditory, olfactory, tactile, gustatory, kinesthetic, and vestibular stimulations. The sessions of stimulations started 4–12 days after the brain lesion. The treatment lasted 1 h and was applied 1–2 times a day. The coma duration and the GCS score were considered. In the second study, Kater (1989) stimulated 30 (traumatic) severely brain-injured patients at least 2 weeks after the brain lesion [23]. The control group was also matched to the experimental group according to the age, the gender, the type of lesion, and the score on the GCS [24]. In both groups, the patients were divided in three subgroups based on the GCS score: deep (GCS 3–6), moderate (GCS 7–10), and light (GCS 11–14). The experimental treatment included the stimulation of six sensory modalities (i.e., visual, auditory, olfactory, tactile, kinesthetic, and verbal). The treatment lasted 45 min and was applied twice a day, 6 days a week during a period of 1–3 months, according to the patient's recovery. A behavioral assessment was performed before and after treatment. These two studies showed a higher recovery in the experimental group than in the control group, suggesting a positive impact of the sensory stimulation programs on the recovery of severely brain-injured patients. The third study conducted by Johnson et al. (1993) included 14 traumatic patients (GCS <8). The experimental group (7 subjects) and the controls group (7 subjects) were matched according to the age and the GCS score [25]. The treatment consisted in stimulating the five senses 20 min a day during the entire stay in the intensive care. GCS scores, brainstem reflexes (e.g., oculo-cephalic and oculo-vestibular reflexes) as well as several physiological measurements (e.g., skin conductance, respiratory and heart rates) were assessed 20 min pre- and posttreatment. However, the authors did not find any significant change.

According to Lombardi et al., these studies do not allow confirming the efficacy of this type of treatment for patients recovering from coma [22]. Indeed, beside an insufficient description of the sensory stimulation program applied, their results are contradictory and their methodology is different (e.g., type and duration of treatment, assessment, and outcome measures), which does not allow the comparison of studies. The authors conclude that there is no reliable evidence supporting the interest of sensory stimulation programs in comatose or vegetative patients. Another bias the authors did not consider is the part of improvements due to spontaneous recovery. Indeed, these studies were mainly performed in the acute or subacute stage, period during which a spontaneous recovery has the highest probability to appear. None of these studies allows dissociating improvements due to the treatment from improvements due to spontaneous recovery.

Since 2002, several studies have been published. They, nevertheless, present the same methodological issues as described above [26–28]. Interestingly, Oh and Seo [28] decided to investigate whether the improvements observed after a sensory stimulation program exceeded spontaneous recovery. The sensory stimulation program involved auditory, visual, olfactory, gustatory, tactile, and kinesthetic stimulations. The consciousness level was assessed by using the GCS scores. An ABA paradigm was used as the treatment was applied during 4 weeks (phase B) and compared to the baselines (phase A). Results showed a significant fluctuation of the behavioral responses according to the presence or the absence of the treatment—more complex responses being observed in the presence of treatment [28]. This study suggests that sensory stimulation programs would have an impact superior to spontaneous recovery on the improvement of consciousness in patients recovering from coma. However, this study included a small number of patients ($n=5$) and was, therefore, mainly descriptive.

Limitations and Perspectives

As regards methodological biases of previous studies, we cannot conclude the effective impact of sensory stimulation programs on the consciousness recovery. It would, therefore, be needed to increase the quality of future studies, e.g., by considering the following points:

The Use of Valid and Sensitive Behavioral Scales

Some of the studies led on the efficacy of sensory stimulation programs do not use valid behavioral scales, but physiological and electrophysiological measurements [22]. However, the detection of physiological and electrophysiological changes is pointless without the observation of clinical and behavioral improvements. The use of a standardized and validated scale detecting such improvements is, therefore, recommended, but is not sufficient as this scale also has to be sensitive. Previous studies have shown that a scale such as the Coma Recovery Scale-Revised [29] allows a better detection of signs of consciousness than the GCS, which is usually used in studies on sensory stimulation programs [30, 31]. The choice of the behavioral scale that will objectify patients' improvements is nevertheless a critical point as it constitutes an indicator of the effectiveness of the treatment.

Studies on Chronic Patients

Future studies should recruit patients being in stable clinical conditions, and therefore beyond the acute stage. Indeed, about 50% of brain-injured patients present a spontaneous recovery during this period [32]. Besides, it is difficult to administer rehabilitation programs in intensive care units where patients are often sedated.

An ABAB Design

This design is one of the oldest and most widely used time-series method developed in behavioral psychology. It typically includes at least one phase of treatment (phase B) alternating with baselines ("non-treatment" phase or phase A). In other words, it allows measuring the effects of treatment as compared to what happens when the treatment is absent or removed, and hence allows comforting that improvements observed are due to the treatment and not to spontaneous recovery. Using such a design may be even more interesting than using a controlled study, as matching patients can be highly problematic as regards the diversity of ages, etiologies, and brain lesions. As mentioned before, this design was successfully used in one study including five patients [28].

Multicentric Studies

The sample size should be sufficient to demonstrate the clinical significance of the treatment. It is, therefore, reasonable to suggest the implementation of multicentric studies in future clinical researches.

Conclusion

Taking care of patients recovering from coma is uneasy, current therapeutics being neither well-developed nor well-validated. Sensory stimulations programs is the most widely known treatment applied to severely brain-injured patients. Until now, no study permitted to demonstrate its clinical interest. Demonstrating the efficacy of treatments is, nevertheless, a necessary step to the improvement of the quality of life of such patients. Further investigations addressing this question are, therefore, needed in the future.

References

1. Wood R. Critical analysis of the concept of sensory stimulation for patients in vegetative states. Brain Inj. 1991;5(4):401–9.
2. Hummel F, Cohen L. Drivers of brain plasticity. Curr Opin Neurol. 2005;18(6):667–74.
3. Voss H, Uluc A, Dyke J, et al. Possible axonal regrowth in late recovery from the minimally conscious state. J Clin Invest. 2006;116(7):2005–11.
4. Jones R, Hux K, Morton-Anderson K, Knepper L. Auditory stimulation effect on a comatose survivor of traumatic brain injury. Arch Phys Med Rehabil. 1994;75(2):164–71.
5. Ansell B, Keenan J. The Western Neuro Sensory Stimulation Profile: a tool for assessing slow-to-recover head-injured patients. Arch Phys Med Rehabil. 1989;70:104–8.
6. Merabet L, Pascual-Leone A. Neural reorganization following sensory loss: the opportunity of change. Nat Rev Neurosci. 2010;11(1):44–52.
7. Barnes S, Finnerty G. Sensory experience and cortical rewiring. Neuroscientist. 2010;16(2): 186–98.
8. Diamond M. Enriching heredity. New York: The Free Press; 1988.
9. Renner M, Rosenzweig M. Enriched and improverished environments: effects on brain and behaviour. New York: Springer; 1987.
10. Nithianantharajah J, Hannan J. Enriched environments, experience-dependent plasticity and disorders of the nervous system. Nat Rev Neurosci. 2006;7(9):697–709.
11. Sale A, Berardi N, Maffei L. Enrich the environment to empower the brain. Trends Neurosci. 2009;32(4):233–9.
12. LeWinn E, Dimancescu M. Environmental deprivation and enrichment in coma. Lancet. 1978;2:156–7.
13. Blackerly WF. Intensity of rehabilitation and length of stay. Brain Inj. 1990;4(2):167–73.
14. Doman G, Wilkinson R, Dimancescu M, Pelligra R. The effects of intense multi-sensory stimulation on coma arousal and recovery. Neuropsych Rehabil. 1993;3(2):203–12.
15. Hall M, MacDonald S, Young G. The effectiveness of directed multisensory stimulation versus non directed stimulation in comatose closed head injured patients: pilot study of a single subject design. Brain Inj. 1992;6(5):435–45.
16. Lippert-Grüner M, Terhaag D. Multimodal early onset stimulation (MEOS) in rehabilitation after brain injury. Brain Inj. 2000;14(6):585–94.
17. Mitchell S, Bradley V, Welch J, Britton P. Coma arousal procedure: a therapeutic intervention in the treatment of head injury. Brain Inj. 1990;4(3):273–9.
18. Sisson R. Effects of auditory stimuli on comatose patients with head injury. Heart Lung. 1990;19(4):373–8.
19. Tablot L, Whitaker H. Brain-injured persons in an altered state of consciousness: measures and intervention strategies. Brain Inj. 1994;8(8):689–99.

20. Wilson S, Powell G, Elliott K, Thwaites H. Sensory stimulation in prolonged coma: four single case studies. Brain Inj. 1991;5(4):393–400.
21. Wilson S, Powell G, Brock D, Thwaites H. Behavioural differences between patients who emerged from vegetative state and those who did not. Brain Inj. 1996;10(7):509–16.
22. Lombardi F. Sensory stimulation of brain-injured individuals in coma or vegetative state: results of a Cochrane systematic review. Clin Rehabil. 2002;16:465–73.
23. Kater K. Response of head-injured patients to sensory stimulation. West J Nurs Res. 1989;11:20–33.
24. Teasdale G, Jennett B. Assessment of coma and impaired consciousness. A practical scale. Lancet. 1974;2(7872):81–4.
25. Johnson D, Roethig Johnston K, Richards D. Biochemical and physiological parameters of recovery in acute severe head injury: responses to multisensory stimulation. Brain Inj. 1993;7(6):491–9.
26. Davis A, Gimenez A. Cognitive-behavioral recovery in comatose patients following auditory sensory stimulation. J Neurosci Nurs. 2003;35(4):202–9.
27. Urbenjaphol P, Jitpanya C, Khaoropthu S. Effects of the sensory stimulation program on recovery in unconscious patients with traumatic brain injury. J Neurosci Nurs. 2009;41:10–6.
28. Oh H, Seo W. Sensory stimulation programme to improve recovery in comatose patients. J Clin Nurs. 2003;12:394–404.
29. Giacino J, Kalmar K, Whyte J. The JFK Coma Recovery Scale-Revised: measurement characteristics and diagnostic utility. Arch Phys Med Rehabil. 2004;85(12):2020–9.
30. Schnakers C, Majerus S, Giacino J, et al. A French validation study of the Coma Recovery Scale-Revised (CRS-R). Brain Inj. 2008;22(10):786–92.
31. Schnakers C, Giacino J, Kalmar K, et al. Does the FOUR score correctly diagnose the vegetative and minimally conscious states? Ann Neurol. 2006;60(6):744–5.
32. Groswasser Z, Cohen M, Blankstein E. Polytrauma associated with traumatic brain injury: incidence, nature and impact on rehabilitation outcome. Brain Inj. 1990;4:161–6.

Chapter 11
Feasibility of Oral Feeding in Patients with Disorders of Consciousness

Audrey Maudoux, Ingrid Breuskin, Olivia Gosseries, Caroline Schnakers, and Audrey Vanhaudenhuyse

Introduction

Eating and drinking are basic pleasures of life, considered as obvious to most of us. However, the ease with which we perform these actions masks the complexity of the underlying neuronal control. Various regions of the central nervous system, from brainstem to cortex, are involved in the realization of this complex sensorimotor sequence. Swallowing involves muscles of the face, tongue, pharynx, larynx, and esophagus, with a total of 26 pairs of muscles, to which must be added the unique

A. Maudoux, M.D. (✉)
Oto-Rhino-Laryngology Head and Neck Surgery Department, University Hospital of Liège, Sart-Tilman-B35, 4000 Liège, Belgium

Coma Science Group, Cyclotron Research Center, University of Liège, Sart-Tilman-B30, 4000 Liège, Belgium
e-mail: amaudoux@doct.ulg.ac.be

I. Breuskin, M.D., Ph.D.
Oto-Rhino-Laryngology Head and Neck Surgery Department, University Hospital of Liège, Sart-Tilman-B35, 4000 Liège, Belgium
e-mail: ibreuskin@alumni.ulg.ac.be

O. Gosseries, M.Sc.
Coma Science Group, Cyclotron Research Center, University of Liège, Sart-Tilman-B30, 4000 Liège, Belgium
e-mail: ogosseries@doct.ulg.ac.be

C. Schnakers, Ph.D. • A. Vanhaudenhuyse, Ph.D.
Coma Science Group, Cyclotron Research Center, University of Liège, Sart-Tilman-B30, 4000 Liège, Belgium
e-mail: c.schnakers@ulg.ac.be; avanhaudenhuyse@ulg.ac.be

C. Schnakers, S. Laureys (eds.), *Coma and Disorders of Consciousness*,
DOI 10.1007/978-1-4471-2440-5_11, © Springer-Verlag London 2012

upper lingual muscle, and five pairs of cranial nerves. The complexity of the underlying neural mechanism as well as the number of muscles and cranial nerves involved made the study of swallowing in animals and humans difficult. Although diagnosis methods, assessment, and rehabilitation of swallowing disorders have been extensively studied, no major breakthrough in the understanding of the neurophysiological basis supporting the phenomenon has been provided. Nevertheless, interest in the study of swallowing has increased in the past few years. Initially, groups of patients with neurological disorders (e.g., stroke) were studied. A precise anatomical study of brain lesions using CT scanner or magnetic resonance imaging (MRI) was correlated with the clinical evaluation of swallowing in order to establish a relationship between neurological injury and the presence and type of dysphagia. Subsequently, the development of functional imaging techniques allowed the study of swallowing in healthy volunteers. According to several studies, the frequency of dysphagia among subjects with severe brain injury varies between 25% and 61% [1–3]. These swallowing difficulties are mainly due to physiological deficits (affecting the swallowing mechanism) and impaired cognition. Faced with the difficult management of patients with altered state of consciousness, the use of gustatory stimuli, as well as the rehabilitation of swallowing could constitute a supplementary therapy which is currently rarely considered [4]. Furthermore, one may ask whether the clinical assessment of swallowing could be used as a tool for neurological diagnosis or prognosis of consciousness recovery. The review presented here aims to summarize our current knowledge regarding the neural control of swallowing (whether initiated voluntarily or not), to assess the role of awareness and willingness on the control of swallowing, and finally, to establish the feasibility of oral feeding in patients with disorders of consciousness.

Neurophysiology of Swallowing

Since Magendie in 1825, swallowing is usually divided into three parts: oral, pharyngeal, and esophageal. The oral phase is usually described as a voluntary phase, the pharyngeal phase and the esophageal phase (which is mainly under the control of the autonomic nervous system) as reflex (Fig. 11.1).

The Oral Phase

The oral phase is the only voluntary stage of swallowing. The different steps of this first phase are the ingestion, mastication, and food insalivation. These steps lead to the formation of the bolus, which will then be transported to the pharynx. During the oral phase, the oral cavity should remain closed in order to contain food. At the front, the contraction of the orbicularis oris muscle acts as the anterior sphincter. At the back, the velum, lowered against the tongue, acts as the posterior sphincter. It prevents the early passage of food in the pharynx. During mastication, the tongue carries food from the teeth to crush, cut, and tear the aliments. The insalivation occurs during chewing. This step has both a digestive role, due to the action of amylase, and a mechanical role

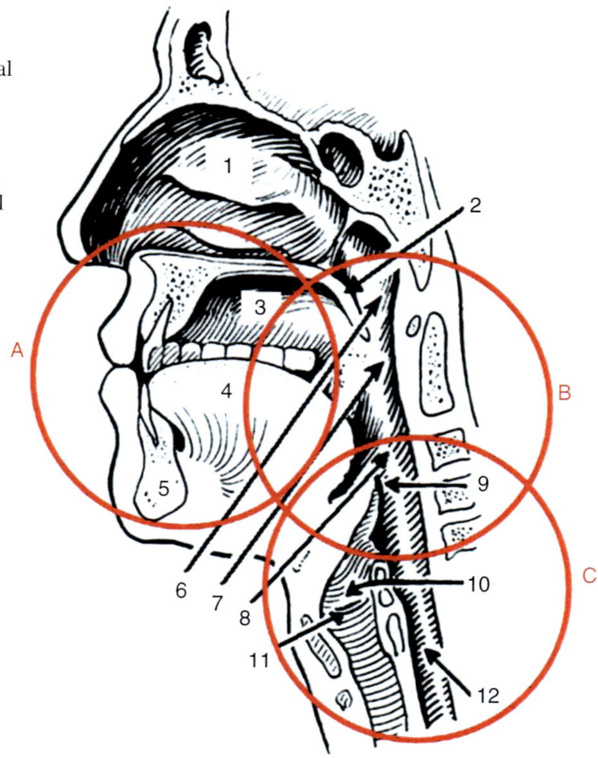

Fig. 11.1 The three phases of swallowing: *A* Oral phase, *B* Pharyngeal phase, *C* Esophageal phase. *1* nasal cavity, *2* soft palate, *3* mouth, *4* tongue, *5* mandible, *6* nasopharynx, *7* oropharynx, *8* laryngopharynx, *9* epiglottis, *10* larynx, *11* vocal cords, *12* esophagus (Adapted from [5])

by providing lubrication and cohesion to the bolus. During the propulsion step, the bolus is moved to the back of the oral cavity. When food reaches the *Wassilieff* area (a mucous membrane covering the soft palate, the root of the tongue, the vallecula, and the posterior pharyngeal wall), the pharyngeal phase of swallowing begins. Thus, the Wassilieff area delimits the transition from the oral phase to the second stage of swallowing—the pharyngeal phase. The oral phase fluctuates in time depending on taste, food consistency, environment, hunger, motivation, and patient's level of consciousness. It relies on good tongue mobility and on perfect function of numerous muscles: the suprahyoid muscles, the jaw closing muscles (temporalis muscle, masseter muscle), the pterygoid and the infrahyoid muscles (allowing stabilization of the hyoid bone), the orbicularis oris muscle, and the palatoglossus muscles.

The Pharyngeal Phase

When the food reaches the pharyngeal space, the swallowing reflex itself starts. This is followed by a series of events leading to the transportation of the bolus to the esophagus and to the protection of the airway. The fine and synchronized movements of the different muscles involved are controlled by the brainstem via the central pattern generator (CPG). This phase includes three stages.

1. *Protection of the nasopharynx and larynx*
   The occlusion of the velopharyngeal sphincter aims to isolate the oropharynx from the nasopharynx. Elevation of the soft palate together with the approximation of the lateral pharyngeal walls avoid nasal reflux of food and liquid. Protection of lower airways is provided by the occlusion of the laryngeal sphincter (elevation of the larynx, closing of the vocal cord plane and of the ventricular folds, forward tilt of the arytenoids, and lowering of the epiglottis). The ascension of the larynx is a critical swallowing step. It protects the airway by positioning the larynx under the root of the tongue and by closing the ventricles of the larynx. This upward movement also promotes the opening of the upper esophageal sphincter (UES).
2. *Propulsion of the bolus through the pharynx*
   The propulsion of the bolus is mainly provided by the posterior movement of the root of the tongue, pushing the bolus into the esophagus. To complete the hypopharyngeal draining, the pharyngeal constrictor muscles contract sequentially, achieving a peristaltic wave and pushing the food bolus from top to bottom.
3. *Upper esophageal sphincter opening*
   During swallowing, the cricopharyngeal muscle relaxes and the sphincter is pulled forward by contraction of suprahyoid muscles, allowing its opening. Finally, the pharyngeal phase ends, and the UES closes until the next swallowing.

The Esophageal Phase

The esophageal phase ensures the transfer of the bolus from the UES to the stomach through a peristaltic wave. By working in sync, the two muscle layers of the esophagus (external longitudinal and inner circular layers) create the movements of peristalsis.

The Neurological Control

Swallowing requires perfect coordination between the different muscles mentioned above. It is achieved through fine control of the central nervous system. Indeed, as the respiratory and digestive tracts cross in the pharynx, the slightest misstep in the sequence of swallowing may cause the passage of part of the bolus into the airway. The main structure in-charge of the neural control is the swallowing CPG, located in the brainstem. The CPG receives both sensory inputs from the periphery (oral cavity, pharynx, and larynx) and cortical afferents. It integrates these informations, develops a motor program, and transmits this program to the motor neuron nuclei. It organizes all the sequential activation of motor neurons involved in swallowing (Fig. 11.2).

The sensory inputs come primarily from the glossopharyngeal (IX) and the superior laryngeal nerves, a branch of the vagus nerve (X), both crucial for airway protection. Stimulation of areas innervated by the glossopharyngeal nerve appears to

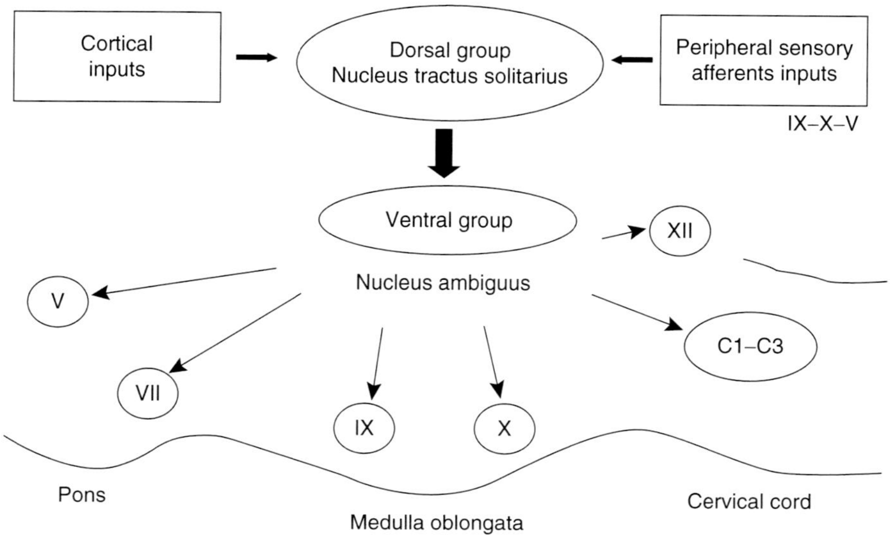

Fig. 11.2 Schematic representation of the central pattern generator (*CPG*). Sensory inputs from the periphery (oral cavity, pharynx, and larynx) and cortical afferents project around the nucleus of the solitary tract (dorsal swallowing group). The dorsal group integrates these informations, develops the motor swallowing program and transmits this program to the premotor neurons of the ventral group, located next to the nucleus ambiguus (Adapted from [6] and [7])

facilitate swallowing in humans [8]. Superior laryngeal nerve stimulation is also efficient to trigger swallowing in most mammals [9]. Informations from the glossopharyngeal and superior laryngeal nerves are transmitted to the swallowing center via the solitary tract. To the sensory inputs coming from the superior laryngeal and glossopharyngeal nerves must be added the influence of sensory afferents from the trigeminal nerve (V), and particularly from one of its branches, the mandibular nerve (V3). Mechanoreceptors located in the oral cavity and at the level of the temporomandibular joints provide informations on the consistency and volume of the bolus. It modulates the motor response by changing its amplitude and/or duration.

In the medulla oblongata, there is a network of interneurons responsible for the development of the motor program of swallowing [6]. This network is divided into two groups: a dorsal group organized at the level of the dorsal solitary nucleus and the reticular formation and a ventral group organized around the nucleus ambiguus. The dorsal cluster receives sensory inputs from the periphery and cortical afferents. It develops the motor program sent to the swallowing motor nuclei by the ventral cluster. The trigeminal motor nuclei are located in the middle part of the pons. They innervate the tensor veli palatini, the anterior belly of digastric, mylohyoid muscles, masseter muscles, temporalis muscles, and medial and lateral pterygoid muscles. The facial motor nuclei are located at the bottom of the pons. They control the muscles of facial expression, the posterior belly of digastric, and stylohyoid muscles. The nucleus ambiguus, which occupies the entire height of the medulla oblongata, controls the innervation of the esophagus and the velopharynx (motor fibers of IX and X) via its rostral part, whereas its caudal part innervates the larynx (the

Table 11.1 Cranial nerves involved in the process of swallowing

Cranial nerves	Role
V Trigeminal Three branches: Ophthalmic nerve (V1) Maxillary nerve (V2) Mandibular nerve (V3)	*Sensory*: face, mouth, cheek, chin, lips, palate, teeth, nasal cavity, mandible, anterior two-thirds of the tongue *Motor:* masticator muscles, tensors of the soft palate, mylohyoid muscles, anterior belly of digastric
VII Facial	*Taste:* two-thirds of the tongue *Secretory:* lacrimal, submandibular, and sublingual glands, mucous membranes of the palate and nose *Motor:* facial expression muscles, nasal muscles, posterior belly of digastric, stylohyoid muscles, stapedius muscles
IX Glossopharyngeal	*Taste:* posterior third of the tongue *Secretory*: parotid glands *Sensory:* posterior third of the tongue, pharynx, and soft palate *Motor:* stylopharyngeus muscle, pharyngeal constrictors
X Vagus	*Taste:* epiglottic region and root of the tongue *Sensory:* epiglottis, laryngeal mucosa *Motor:* esophageal muscles, laryngeal muscles (except stylopharyngeus) with the help of the accessory nerve (XI), muscles of the soft palate (except tensor veli palatini)
XII Hypoglossal	*Motor:* all the muscles of the tongue (except palatoglossus), geniohyoid muscles, thyrohyoid muscles

Adapted from [5, 10, 11]

bulbar accessory nerve [XI]). The hypoglossal nuclei (XII) associated with the C1 roots innervates the muscles of the tongue. The C2 and C3 cervical roots, together with the hypoglossal nerves, control the infrahyoid muscles.

In summary, sensory informations are dependent on three pairs of cranial nerves: the trigeminal (V), the glossopharyngeal (IX), and the vagus nerves (X). Yet, afferents from the superior laryngeal nerve are the most powerful to trigger swallowing. The innervation of the different muscles involved in swallowing is, in turn, provided by five pairs of cranial nerves: the trigeminal (V), the facial (VII), the glossopharyngeal (IX), the vagus (X), and the hypoglossal nerves (XII) (Table 11.1).

Swallowing and Consciousness

Animal Studies

At the beginning of the last century, Sherrington observed swallowing in decerebrate cats, in which regions located above the pons were disconnected from the brainstem [12]. He described the effects of different stimuli (electrical, mechanical, liquid, or chemical) which, in contact with a region innervated by the superior laryngeal nerve, could trigger swallowing. This swallowing, neither involving oral preparation nor propulsion of the bolus, was regarded as reflex. The swallowing movement observed in Sherrington's cats can be divided into three stages: the closure of the larynx, the propulsion of the bolus into the esophagus, and the opening of the UES [13]. These three steps involve structures innervated by cranial nerves V, VII, X, and the cervical plexus, C1–C3, whose nuclei are distributed in the lower brainstem and spinal cord. Swallowing reflex has also been observed in decerebrate and anesthetized goats. Swallowing was triggered by electrical stimulation of the superior laryngeal nerve [14]. When trying to reproduce the experiment with glossopharyngeal nerve electrical stimulation, no swallowing reflex was observed. However, it seemed to have a facilitating role on the swallowing movements induced by the stimulation of the superior laryngeal nerve. These experiments suggest that triggering swallowing movements in decerebrate mammals are possible, even in the absence of a cortical control.

Human Studies

Ultrasound studies on oral sensorimotor function and swallowing in human fetuses showed early onset of swallowing mechanisms [15]. Indeed, the swallowing is important for regulating the volume and composition of the amniotic fluid. The pharyngeal phase of swallowing is one of the first pharyngeal motor responses observed in fetuses and appears between the 10th and 14th week of gestation. The growing network of interneurons in the brainstem controlling the pharyngeal phase of swallowing achieved a functional level during fetal development as early as the 11th week. From the 22nd to 24th weeks of gestation, swallowing movements are constantly observed. The swallowing reflex seems also present even in the absence of cortex in the human fetus. Indeed, several ultrasound studies show the presence of swallowing movements in anencephalic fetuses [16]. These observations demonstrate that human fetus can achieve swallowing movements even before a complete development of cortical and subcortical structures. One might conclude that in humans, as observed in other mammals, swallowing seems to be mainly controlled by the brainstem. However, many electrophysiological studies, neuroimaging, and clinical observations show that the cerebral cortex also plays an important role in the process of swallowing [17–19], even when the swallowing is considered as reflex or automatic [20, 21]. This cortical involvement becomes evident when looking at the incidence of dysphagia among subjects suffering from stroke. In these patients, with anoxic brain damage, rate of dysphagia ranges from <30% [22] to more than 50% [23]. Thus, lesions of the cerebral cortex have important implications on human swallowing. Since the early studies of cortical electrical stimulation done by Penfield, the involvement of the cerebral cortex in the process of swallowing has been confirmed. Through the use of transcranial magnetic stimulation (TMS), Hamdy and colleagues demonstrated the existence of an asymmetrical somatotopic representation of the different muscles involved in swallowing [24], which was not correlated to the laterality of the subject. If during a stroke the hemisphere with the largest representation of the corticospinal tract involved in swallowing is damage, it increases the risk of dysphagia [24]. Recovery of an effective swallowing function, in the case of unilateral involvement of the corticospinal tract, depends on the presence and development of the same tract in the contralateral hemisphere [25–27]. The development of functional imaging techniques (Positron Emission Tomography: PET, functional magnetic resonance imaging: fMRI) has revolutionized the study of the brain. These techniques allowed for a better understanding of cortical mechanisms involved in swallowing and confirm the important role of the cerebral cortex. The main cortical and subcortical areas involved are the cerebellum, the basal ganglia and the sensorimotor, prefrontal, anterior cingulate, insula, and temporoparietal regions [28–32].

Precentral Gyrus

The precentral gyrus is the most consistently cited region in functional imaging studies exploring swallowing. It encompasses the premotor cortex (including the supplementary motor area, SMA) and the primary motor cortex. This region controls the muscles of the oral cavity, pharynx, and larynx [24] and is mainly involved in planned and voluntary movements. However, the precentral gyrus seems also active during the production of automatic swallowing and its role in the realization automatic movement has to be clarified [20]. The SMA is located in front of the primary motor cortex. This region is related to the planning of complex movements and especially sequential movements. It seems to have a modulatory action on the motor sequence and to be involved in the initiation of the pharygo-oesophageal phase of swallowing [28].

The Prefrontal Cortex

The prefrontal cortex is the anterior part of the frontal lobe and is located in front of the premotor areas. This region is associated with the planning of complex cognitive tasks. It is involved in the genesis of emotional states and in the regulation of autonomic changes accompanying those states. The prefrontal cortex is also implicated in the analysis of olfactory information.

The Anterior Cingulate Cortex

The anterior cingulate cortex is important for conscious awareness and for the processing of stimuli related to emotion. Activation of the anterior cingulate cortex could account for the affective and attentional aspect of swallowing. Others consider this region (which is involved in cognitive and attentional processes) as an interface between intention and execution of the motor sequences involved in swallowing [33]. In addition, the anterior cingulate cortex also plays a role in mediating the visceral motor responses of the digestive tract.

The Insula

Several functional neuroimaging studies report activation of the insula during swallowing [20, 28, 34]. Damage to this isolated region may induce dysphagia [34]. The insula is involved, among other regions, in monitoring and analyzing informations concerning the body's homeostatic state. It is also involved in visceral motor control (automatic) [35], somatic sensations of the orofacial region in primates, voluntary control of orofacial movements, and control of speech. Activation of the insula seems to play a role in integrating the sensory and motor aspects of the digestive tract.

Parietal Regions and the Postcentral Gyrus

The sensory cortex is involved in the processing of facial as well as gustatory stimuli [36]. Its activation during swallowing reflects the large number of sensory informations coming from the oropharyngeal region. As already discussed, the sensory inputs are essential for the regulation of swallowing [20].

Temporal Regions

In their work, Martin and colleagues proposed to link the temporal cortex activation, more exactly the primary auditory cortex, to the analysis of acoustic stimuli produced by chewing and swallowing [20]. Indeed, we receive, via bone conduction, sounds associated with swallowing. Furthermore, a study using PET suggested the involvement of the anteromedial portion of the temporal lobe in the recognition of gustatory stimuli [37].

The Basal Ganglia

The basal ganglia encompass several subcortical structures such as the caudate nucleus, putamen or globus pallidus. These structures receive information from various brain areas (frontal, prefrontal, and parietal) and transmit them to the SMA. In doing so, the basal ganglia exert a facilitator effect on movement. Clinical studies show that lesions of the basal ganglia, as found in Parkinson's disease, lead to difficulty in coordinating the oropharyngeal phase of swallowing.

The Cerebellum

The cerebellum is known to be a regulator of the motor sequence [38–40]. It integrates the sensory inputs and organizes, based on these inputs, the efferent motor response [41]. It ensures a correct pharyngeal and laryngeal synergy and chronometry such as elevating the larynx, closing the glottis, or triggering the swallowing reflex.

The fact that many different cortical areas are activated during swallowing is not surprising. Indeed, most studies are based on observation of the mechanisms involved during voluntary swallowing (i.e., the swallowing of food or saliva on command). Unlike voluntary swallowing, one might think that spontaneous swallowing might not require cortical control. However, observation of patients with swallowing apraxia suggests the opposite. This disorder—characterized by the inability to perform reflex swallowing while voluntary swallowing (i.e., swallowing on command) is preserved—was observed in some patients with left frontolateral cortical lesions [42]. In addition, several studies have shown that reflex swallowing is associated with activation of several brain areas [20, 21]. The network activated during this particular type of swallowing is different from that observed during voluntary swallowing. According to Kern et al., reflex swallowing activates the primary sensorimotor cortex in contrast to voluntary swallowing, which activates, in addition to this region, a multitude of other cortical regions such as the insula, prefrontal and cingulate gyri, cuneus, and precuneus [21]. These additional regions could reflect the preparation and the voluntary realization of the movement. Another study of Martin and colleagues showed a higher activity of the posterior part (caudal part) of the anterior cingulate gyrus during voluntary swallowing as opposed to reflex swallowing [20]. Although studies on decerebrated animals show that stimulation of laryngeal or pharyngeal mucosa may trigger a swallowing reflex movement without any cortical control, studies in adult humans show that cortical activity is needed both in voluntary and swallowing reflex. A certain level of cortical integrity seems necessary for the realization of voluntary or swallowing reflex movements. However, the impact of the level of consciousness on a patient's swallowing ability has to be determined. The observation of swallowing in different physiological alteration of consciousness states (e.g., during sleep), or under medication (e.g., during anesthesia) could give us interesting clue. During sleep, swallowing movements are less frequent and long periods without swallowing are observed. When swallowing occurs, it is associated with signs of awakenings on electroencephalography (EEG), both during REM (rapid eye movement) and non-REM sleep. Moreover, the frequency of swallowing movements seems related to the stage of sleep. When sleep deepens, less swallowing movements are observed [43, 44]. In patients receiving general anesthesia, changes in swallowing reflex are often observed during the perioperative period. Several reasons can explain this swallowing alteration: traumatic reasons (i.e., mucosal lesions as a consequence of endotracheal intubation) and pharmacological reasons associated to the own pharmacodynamic effects of each anesthetic agent used, including alteration of consciousness [45].

Oral Feeding in Patients with Disorder of Consciousness

Although approaches aiming at improving the well-being of patients with disorder of consciousness increase, and although the use of sensory stimuli are used more and more often in rehabilitation programs, the use of oral and gustatory stimuli appears to have been shelved. In this challenging population, the utility of gustatory stimuli is difficult to address. Indeed, the frequency of swallowing disorders associated with traumatic or anoxic brain injury varies between 25% and 61% [1–3]. In addition, repeated inhalation can lead to complications (e.g., aspiration pneumonia) with dramatic consequences in this fragile population. Unresponsive wakefulness syndrome (UWS) patients are characterized by a lack of wakefulness and awareness. They only show reflexive movements. From an anatomical point of view, their brainstem is relatively preserved, while the white and gray matters are severely affected. They also show an impairment of their associative cortices involved in the realization of complex information processing such as memory, attention, planning, or language. Unlike UWS patients, minimally conscious state (MCS) patients show reproducible but fluctuating signs of consciousness (e.g., visual tracking or response to command). These MCS patients are, however, not able to communicate [46]. Their brain metabolic activity is higher than in UWS patients [47] and their associative areas are less affected. Based on our current knowledge, we know that relative preservation of the brainstem, as observed in UWS patients, cannot guarantee the absence of a swallowing disorder. We also know that the cerebral cortex plays an important role in either voluntary or reflex swallowing [20]. Accordingly, given the better overall brain activity in MCS patients, the probability of observing a preserved swallowing function with a low aspiration risk (i.e., with a low risk of penetration of ingested material in the airway), is theoretically more important than in UWS patients. However, any cortical lesion, even if limited, is likely to cause major swallowing disorders.

According to a study of MacKay and colleagues conducted in patients with traumatic brain injury, in whom 41% showed signs of aspiration, the factor influencing the most the recovery of a full oral feeding was the *Ranchos Los Amigos (RLA)* score [48]. This scale was developed at Ranchos Los Amigos Hospital in California to assess cognitive functioning [49]. A score lower than III on the RLA scale refers to an UWS patient, a score between III and V to a MCS patient, and a score of VI to a patient who emerged from the minimally conscious state. In the MacKay study, the minimal RLA score required to be able to begin an oral therapy was IV. To achieve a complete diet of three meals a day, a score of VI or higher was required. According to this study, the patient's ability to eat seemed related to the level of consciousness. For these authors, the severity of the swallowing disorders is related to a low score on the *Glasgow coma scale (GCS)*, a low RLA score, the presence of a tracheotomy, and at least 2 weeks of mechanical ventilation [1]. Similarly, Ward and colleagues observed that patients with a GCS score between 3 and 8 showed a longer delay before the resumption of oral feeding compared to patients with a GCS score above 8 [50]. Other studies also show that low level of consciousness is associated with low oral feeding capacity [51, 52]. To assess the feasibility of an effective and objective evaluation of swallowing in patients with severe disorders of consciousness, Pirozzi and colleagues evaluated 12 tracheotomized patients with severe disorder of consciousness following a traumatic brain injury [53]. In this study, one of the secondary objectives was to evaluate the feasibility of using liquid or solid food in a sensory stimulation program at the acute phase. Out of the 12 subjects, 7 were diagnosed as UWS (RLA score of II) and 5 as MCS (RLA score of III). First, for 92% of their patients, a comprehensive swallowing assessment including video-fluoroscopy (using four substances of different consistencies) could be achieved. Video-fluoroscopy involves the ingestion of a barium-based contrast. The progression and distribution of this product in the oral cavity, pharynx, and esophagus are then followed using an X-ray system, allowing the observation and evaluation of the three phases of swallowing. Thus, no matter the level of consciousness, it seems possible to objectively assess the patient's swallowing abilities. It should be noted that the authors have reported signs of aspiration in 25% of their subjects ($n=3$), which is less than the aspiration rate reported by MacKay and colleagues [1]. In these three patients, two were UWS and presented lesions in the brainstem and cortex. The third was MCS and had only cortical lesions. All the aspirations observed in these three patients were silent (i.e., occurring without visible or audible sign such as a cough reflex). In consequence, traditional bedside swallowing assessments would have missed aspirations in these three patients. This corroborates previous publications showing that traditional clinical bedside swallowing assessments are only 66% accurate in screening aspiration risks [54, 55]. Making a decision on whether oral feeding can be safely resumed cannot be done based on bedside evaluation alone. Besides swallowing assessment, the authors performed various exercises with the patients. Their rehabilitation technique for oral feeding included oral range of motion exercises, thermal and taste stimulations with small amounts of specified food, and/or drink consistencies, therapy to reduce bite reflex and caregiver education. Following this therapy, none of the patients developed aspiration pneumonia. When discharged from the acute care, all subjects were receiving some amount of food and/or drink. Moreover, gastrostomy could be withdrawn in five subjects as oral feeding was sufficient to meet their daily needs. An improvement in cognitive-behavioral functions was also observed in 10 out of 12 subjects (6 UWS and 4 MCS). They had an RLA score of III–VII at the time of discharge. Again, the patient's swallowing abilities seem to be related to changes in the patient's level of consciousness, at least during the acute phase. However, it is impossible to determine whether the increase of oral feeding could be related to the rehabilitation effect or to the spontaneous evolution of consciousness. Similarly, Brady and colleagues [4] have evaluated 25 patients with altered state of consciousness with an RLA score varying between II and III (UWS and MCS). These patients were divided into two groups: one group of 10 subjects with an RLA score of III who received oral feeding rapidly and a second group of 15 subjects for whom the initiation of oral feeding was delayed. In this second group, feeding was started as soon as an RLA score of III or more was reached. For all these patients, an objective swallowing assessment was performed either by using video-fluoroscopy or fiberoptic endoscopic evaluation. None of the patient showed evidence of inhalation during the evaluation and none of the patient with an RLA score lower than III received oral feeding. At discharge, when considering the number of patients receiving three oral meals a day, there was no difference between the two groups. Again, this study highlights the fact that patients with an altered state of consciousness can fully participate in objective swallowing assessments. For the authors, oral feeding is related to consciousness. On the contrary, there seems to be no relationship between early therapeutic oral feeding and improvement of consciousness. They concluded that it is safe to provide therapeutic oral feeding (i.e., small amounts of food given by a speech therapist) to patients with an RLA score of III (MCS) under specific conditions. These conditions are: no demonstration of aspiration or elimination of aspiration by means of volume or consistency modification (on a baseline instrumental swallowing examination) and close supervision during oral feeding.

Conclusions

Swallowing is a complex sensorimotor function divided into three phases: oral, pharyngeal, and oesophageal. The achievement of the complete swallowing sequence involves the muscles of the face, tongue, pharynx, larynx, and esophagus, with a total of 26 pairs of muscles, to which must be added the unique upper lingual muscle and five pairs of cranial nerves. Various regions of the central nervous system, from brainstem to cortex, are involved in the realization of this complex sensorimotor sequence. Because the respiratory and digestive tracts cross in the pharynx, the slightest misstep in the sequence of swallowing may lead to complications sometimes life-threatening. The study of the neurophysiology of swallowing has evolved since the late nineteenth century and Penfield's studies, using direct electrical brain stimulation, to the most recent studies using TMS, PET, and fMRI. Initially, researches focused on the study of peripheral nerves, the organization of the CPG, and the importance of the brainstem. Later, they focused on the involvement of cortical and subcortical regions in reflex and voluntary swallowing movement, and the interactions between these cortical regions and the CPG.

Dysphagia concerns more than half of the patients with severe brain injury [1] and only a few UWS and MCS patients receive oral feeding. We know that swallowing is controlled by a region located in the brainstem, the CPG, which incorporates the afferents from the periphery in order to select the best motor response. We also know that for both voluntary and reflex swallowing, cortical and subcortical brain structures are involved. Only a few studies focused on swallowing disorders in patients with impaired consciousness. However, all tend to state that the level of consciousness during the acute phase determines the feasibility of resuming oral feeding [1, 4, 48, 50–52]. Similarly, rapid resumption of oral feeding in patients with altered state of consciousness is considered as a sign of better prognosis [56]. This is true in the acute phase and it would be interesting to evaluate whether a relationship between consciousness and oral feeding still exists in the chronic phase.

Conversely, the use of therapeutic oral feeding does not appear to affect the recovery of consciousness [4]. Thus, rehabilitation of swallowing should not be considered as a therapeutic tool but rather as a management option for these patients. Including the rehabilitation of swallowing as part of a more global sensory stimulation program could be achieved in this particular population and improve patient's quality of life. Indeed, administration of a therapeutic oral feeding in selected patients (with RLA score III [MCS]), seems safe [4]. Because of the limited number of studies that have addressed this issue and because those studies included only few patients, it is difficult to give a clear and definitive answer to our initial questions. Further studies have to be performed in a larger sample of patients and have to evaluate the relationship between consciousness recovery, lesions of the central nervous system, and swallowing abilities, both during acute and chronic phase. In conclusion, the evaluation of swallowing abilities is important and should be a part of the evaluation of all patients with altered state of consciousness. Indeed, whatever the underlying neurological disease, dysphagia, because of its potential respiratory and nutritional complications, is a marker of poor prognosis.

References

1. Mackay LE, Morgan AS, Bernstein BA. Factors affecting oral feeding with severe traumatic brain injury. J Head Trauma Rehabil. 1999;14:435–47.
2. Winstein CJ. Neurogenic dysphagia. Frequency, progression, and outcome in adults following head injury. Phys Ther. 1983;63:1992–7.
3. Mackay LE, Morgan AS, Bernstein BA. Swallowing disorders in severe brain injury: risk factors affecting return to oral intake. Arch Phys Med Rehabil. 1999;80:365–71.
4. Brady SL, Darragh M, Escobar NG, et al. Persons with disorders of consciousness: are oral feedings safe/effective? Brain Inj. 2006;20:1329–34.
5. Bleeckx, D. Dysphagie: évaluation et rééducation des troubles de la déglutition. De Boeck 2002, 1st edn.
6. Jean A. Brain stem control of swallowing: neuronal network and cellular mechanisms. Physiol Rev. 2001;81:929–69.
7. Ertekin C, Aydogdu I. Neurophysiology of swallowing. Clin Neurophysiol. 2003;114:2226–44.
8. Sinclair WJ. Initiation of reflex swallowing from the naso- and oropharynx. Am J Physiol. 1970;218:956–60.
9. Doty R. Neural organisation of deglutition. In: Code CF, editor. Handbook of physiology. Washington, DC: American Physiological Society; 1968. p. 1861–902.
10. McFarland. L'anatomie en orthophonie : Parole, voix et déglutition. Elsevier Masson 2006.
11. Mistry S, Hamdy S. Neural control of feeding and swallowing. Phys Med Rehabil Clin N Am. 2008;19:709–28, vii-viii.
12. Miller FR, Sherrington CS. Some observations on the buccopharyngeal stage of reflex deglutition in the cat. Q J Exp Physiol. 1916;9:147–86.
13. Hughes T. Neurology of swallowing and oral feeding disorders: assessment and management. J Neurol Neurosurg Psychiatry. 2003;74 Suppl 3:iii48–52.
14. Ciampini G, Jean A. Role of glossopharyngeal and trigeminal afferents in the initiation and propagation of swallowing. I–Glossopharyngeal afferents. J Physiol Paris. 1980;76:49–60.
15. Delaney AL, Arvedson JC. Development of swallowing and feeding: prenatal through first year of life. Dev Disabil Res Rev. 2008;14:105–17.

16. Peleg D, Goldman JA. Fetal deglutition: a study of the anencephalic fetus. Eur J Obstet Gynecol Reprod Biol. 1978;8:133–6.
17. Martin RE, Sessle BJ. The role of the cerebral cortex in swallowing. Dysphagia. 1993;8:195–202.
18. Miller AJ. The neuroscientific principles of swallowing and dysphagia. San Diego/London: Singular Publication Group; 1999.
19. Michou E, Hamdy S. Cortical input in control of swallowing. Curr Opin Otolaryngol Head Neck Surg. 2009;17:166–71.
20. Martin RE, Goodyear BG, Gati JS, Menon RS. Cerebral cortical representation of automatic and volitional swallowing in humans. J Neurophysiol. 2001;85:938–50.
21. Kern MK, Jaradeh S, Arndorfer RC, Shaker R. Cerebral cortical representation of reflexive and volitional swallowing in humans. Am J Physiol Gastrointest Liver Physiol. 2001; 280:G354–60.
22. Young EC, Durant-Jones L. Developing a dysphagia program in an acute care hospital: a needs assessment. Dysphagia. 1990;5:159–65.
23. Gordon C, Hewer RL, Wade DT. Dysphagia in acute stroke. Br Med J (Clin Res Ed). 1987;295:411–4.
24. Hamdy S, Aziz Q, Rothwell JC, et al. The cortical topography of human swallowing musculature in health and disease. Nat Med. 1996;2:1217–24.
25. Hamdy S, Aziz Q, Rothwell JC, et al. Explaining oropharyngeal dysphagia after unilateral hemispheric stroke. Lancet. 1997;350:686–92.
26. Hamdy S, Rothwell JC, Aziz Q, et al. Long-term reorganization of human motor cortex driven by short-term sensory stimulation. Nat Neurosci. 1998;1:64–8.
27. Hamdy S, Aziz Q, Rothwell JC, et al. Recovery of swallowing after dysphagic stroke relates to functional reorganization in the intact motor cortex. Gastroenterology. 1998;115:1104–12.
28. Hamdy S, Mikulis DJ, Crawley A, et al. Cortical activation during human volitional swallowing: an event-related fMRI study. Am J Physiol. 1999;277:G219–25.
29. Hamdy S, Rothwell JC, Brooks DJ, et al. Identification of the cerebral loci processing human swallowing with H2(15)O PET activation. J Neurophysiol. 1999;81:1917–26.
30. Mosier K, Patel R, Liu WC, et al. Cortical representation of swallowing in normal adults: functional implications. Laryngoscope. 1999;109:1417–23.
31. Zald DH, Pardo JV. The functional neuroanatomy of voluntary swallowing. Ann Neurol. 1999;46:281–6.
32. Mosier KM, Liu WC, Maldjian JA, Shah R, Modi B. Lateralization of cortical function in swallowing: a functional MR imaging study. AJNR Am J Neuroradiol. 1999;20:1520–6.
33. Paus T. Primate anterior cingulate cortex: where motor control, drive and cognition interface. Nat Rev Neurosci. 2001;2:417–24.
34. Daniels SK, Foundas AL. The role of the insular cortex in dysphagia. Dysphagia. 1997;12:146–56.
35. Penfield W, Rasmussen T. The cerebral cortex of man. New York: Macmillan; 1950.
36. Burton H, Benjamin RM. Central projections of the gustatory system. In: Beidler LM, editor. Handbook of sensory physiology, Chemical Senses Sect 2, Taste, vol. 4. Berlin: Springer; 1971. p. 148–63.
37. Small DM, Jones-Gotman M, Zatorre RJ, et al. A role for the right anterior temporal lobe in taste quality recognition. J Neurosci. 1997;17:5136–42.
38. Miall RC. The cerebellum, predictive control and motor coordination. Novartis Found Symp. 1998;218:272–84; discussion 84–90.
39. Ivry R. Cerebellar timing systems. Int Rev Neurobiol. 1997;41:555–73.
40. Doya K. Complementary roles of basal ganglia and cerebellum in learning and motor control. Curr Opin Neurobiol. 2000;10:732–9.
41. Hikosaka O, Nakahara H, Rand MK, et al. Parallel neural networks for learning sequential procedures. Trends Neurosci. 1999;22:464–71.
42. Robbins J, Levin RL. Swallowing after unilateral stroke of the cerebral cortex: preliminary experience. Dysphagia. 1988;3:11–7.

43. Lichter I, Muir RC. The pattern of swallowing during sleep. Electroencephalogr Clin Neurophysiol. 1975;38:427–32.
44. Sato K, Nakashima T. Human adult deglutition during sleep. Ann Otol Rhinol Laryngol. 2006;115:334–9.
45. de Larminat V, Dureuil B. Changes in the deglutition reflex during the perioperative period. Ann Fr Anesth Reanim. 1994;13:49–56.
46. Giacino JT, Ashwal S, Childs N, et al. The minimally conscious state: definition and diagnostic criteria. Neurology. 2002;58:349–53.
47. Laureys S, Owen AM, Schiff ND. Brain function in coma, vegetative state, and related disorders. Lancet Neurol. 2004;3:537–46.
48. MacKay LaM AS. Early swallowing disorders with severe head injuries: relationships between the RLA and the progression of oral intake. Dysphagia. 1993;8:161.
49. Hagen C. The Rancho Levels of Cognitive Functioning. The revised levels - 3rd edition. 1998. Rancho Los Amigos Medical Center.
50. Ward EC, Green K, Morton AL. Patterns and predictors of swallowing resolution following adult traumatic brain injury. J Head Trauma Rehabil. 2007;22:184–91.
51. Cherney LR, Halper AS. Swallowing problems in adults with traumatic brain injury. Semin Neurol. 1996;16:349–53.
52. Morgan A, Ward E, Murdoch B, et al. Incidence, characteristics, and predictive factors for Dysphagia after pediatric traumatic brain injury. J Head Trauma Rehabil. 2003;18:239–51.
53. O'Neil-Pirozzi TM, Momose KJ, Mello J, et al. Feasibility of swallowing interventions for tracheostomized individuals with severely disordered consciousness following traumatic brain injury. Brain Inj. 2003;17:389–99.
54. Splaingard ML, Hutchins B, Sulton LD, Chaudhuri G. Aspiration in rehabilitation patients: videofluoroscopy vs bedside clinical assessment. Arch Phys Med Rehabil. 1988;69:637–40.
55. Linden P, Kuhlemeier KV, Patterson C. The probability of correctly predicting subglottic penetration from clinical observations. Dysphagia. 1993;8:170–9.
56. Formisano R, Voogt RD, Buzzi MG, et al. Time interval of oral feeding recovery as a prognostic factor in severe traumatic brain injury. Brain Inj. 2004;18:103–9.

Chapter 12
Pharmacological Treatments

Olivia Gosseries, Marie Thonnard, and Steven Laureys

Introduction

Disorders of consciousness (DOC) resulting from a severe brain injury include coma [1], the vegetative state [2], and the minimally conscious state [3]. Coma is characterized by a complete absence of arousal and awareness whereas the vegetative state is characterized by an absence of clinical signs of consciousness in spite of a preserved vigilance (opening of the eyes). Patients in a minimally conscious state (MCS) show some signs of consciousness (such as nonreflexive movements without language comprehension, MCS−; or such as command following, MCS+) [4] but remain unable to communicate. If consciousness disorders are currently more clearly defined, no pharmacological treatment is known to improve the level of consciousness of these patients as demonstrated by placebo controlled randomized studies. Evidence based recommendations cannot be provided because there are only a few uncontrolled studies that are often methodologically suboptimal [5]. Pilot studies and case reports showed that some severely brain-damaged patients

O. Gosseries, M.Sc. (✉)
Coma Science Group, Cyclotron Research Centre, University of Liège,
Allée du 6 août, Sart Tilman B30, 4000 Liège, Belgium

Department of Neurology, University Hospital of Liège,
Liège, Belgium

National Fund for Scientific Research,
Liège, Belgium
e-mail: ogosseries@doct.ulg.ac.be

M. Thonnard, M.Sc. • S. Laureys, M.D., Ph.D.
Coma Science Group, Cyclotron Research Centre, University of Liège,
Allée du 6 août, Sart Tilman B30, 4000 Liège, Belgium

Department of Neurology, University Hospital of Liège,
Liège, Belgium
e-mail: marie.thonnard@ulg.ac.be; steven.laureys@ulg.ac.be

C. Schnakers, S. Laureys (eds.), *Coma and Disorders of Consciousness*,
DOI 10.1007/978-1-4471-2440-5_12, © Springer-Verlag London 2012

could benefit from pharmacological, rehabilitation, or sensory stimulation treatments; but, in general, responses to treatment still remain unsatisfactory.

Several pharmacological agents can contribute to the recovery of consciousness in some patients with an altered state of consciousness by targeting various pathways of the central nervous system. Sensory perception is controlled by a complex neural network, which includes reticulothalamic cholinergic projections, thalamocortical, and reticulocortical glutaminergic projections. Lesions in the white matter connections of these networks may affect consciousness and cognition, and several drugs including dopaminergic agents can act on this network by supporting a recovery of consciousness.

This chapter summarizes the current state of knowledge on potentially useful drugs acting on the recovery of consciousness in severely brain-damaged patients and provides indications on the underlying mechanisms possibly explaining the effects of these drugs on the awakening and recovery of consciousness. Exploratory and retrospective studies as well as case reports concerning sporadic cases of spectacular recovery will be discussed regarding drugs as amantadine, levodopa, bromocriptine, apomorphine, methyphenidate, zolpidem, baclofen, sertaline, amitriptyline, desipramine, and lamotrigine (Table 12.1).

Potential Pharmacological Treatments

Amantadine

Amantadine is an old dopaminergic agent initially used in the treatment of Parkinson's disease. For its antiviral properties, amantadine was also employed against influenza. It increases the availability of dopamine in the striatum both at the pre- and postsynaptic levels, facilitates the release of dopamine, and delays its recapture, resulting in an increase of synaptic dopamine concentration. At the postsynaptic level, amantadine increases the number of dopaminergic receptors [6]. It is also a dose-dependent antagonist of the *N*-methyl-D-aspartate receptors.

The use of amantadine is correlated with a better outcome among severe traumatic brain-injured patients. A retrospective study has shown, e.g., that in 74 acute traumatic patients diagnosed in a vegetative state, the group treated with amantadine ($n=41$) obtained higher scores on the Glasgow Coma Scale (GCS) [7] when discharged from the intensive care unit than the group who did not receive the drug [8]. Mortality was also lower in the treatment group (6%) than in the nontreatment group (51%) [8]. Another study on 35 patients showed improvement of behavioral scores (mini-mental state examination [MMSE] [9], Glasgow outcome scale [10], and disability rating scale [DRS] [11]) during a treatment over 6 weeks in the acute phase of severe traumatic brain injury [12]. Note that these two studies took place when the patients were in acute stage and, thus, presented a bias of spontaneous recovery, which may have interfered with

Table 12.1 Pharmacological treatment studies aiming to improve the level of consciousness in patients with severe brain damage with chronic disorders of consciousness

Pharmacological agent	Study (first author, year)	*N*/etiol.	Diagnostic	Interval lesion-treatment	Treatment	Effect	Results	Type of study	Ref
Dopaminergic agent									
Amantadine	Schnakers (2008)	1anox	MCS	2 years	200 mg/day for 6 weeks	+	↑ CRS-R score, response to command, automatic motor behavior	Prospective, ABAB paradigm	[16]
	Patrick (2006)	10TBI	VS/MCS	>1 month	50 mg/day for 3 weeks, 100 mg/day for 1 week, 50 mg/day for 2 weeks	+	↑ CNC, WNSSP, DRS scores	Prospective, double-blind randomized	[19]
	Hughes (2005)	123TBI	Severe lesion	±6 weeks	2 × 100 mg for 1 week, 200 mg 2×/day for 2 weeks	/	No improvement	Retrospective	[20]
	Saniova (2004)	41TBI	VS	<3 months	200 mg 2×/day for 3 days	+	↑ GCS score, ↓ mortality	Retrospective	[8]
	Meythaler (2002)	35TBI	MCS	4 days to 6 weeks	200 mg/day for 6 weeks	+	↑ MMSE, GOS, DRS scores	Prospective, placebo controlled double-blind randomized	[12]
	Zafonte (1998)	1TBI	MCS	5 months	100 mg/day, ↑100 mg/5 days with maximum 400 mg/day. After 35 days, diminution 100 mg/5 days, when 100 mg/day, ↑ again	+	Emergence of MCS, ↑ CNC score, active participation	Case-study, ABAB paradigm	[14]
	Gualtieri (1989)	30TBI	Moderate to severe lesion	2–144 months	50–100 mg/day, ↑ 50–100 mg/week during 6 weeks up to 1 year. If no response, stop treatment after 6 weeks	+	↑ awakening, ↓ tiredness, ↓ distractedness and ↓ aggressiveness	Case-study	[17]

(continued)

Table 12.1 (continued)

Pharmacological agent	Study (first author, year)	*N*/etiol.	Diagnostic	Interval lesion-treatment	Treatment	Effect	Results	Type of study	Ref
Levodopa	Matsuda (2005)	5TBI	VS/MCS	3–22 months	Up to 450 mg/day	+	Emergence from VS and MCS, response to command, verbal and written production, functional communication	Case-study	[24]
	Krimchansky (2004)	8TBI	VS	1–7 months	5/250 mg (carbidopa), 25% of a tablet 3×/day, ↑ of a quarter of tablet every week. Maximum three tablets/day	+	Response to command within 2 weeks, functional communication within 1 month, one patient remains MCS	Prospective	[25]
	Matsuda (2003)	3TBI	VS	3–12 months	100/25 mg (carbidopa) 2–3×/day	+	Response to command, visual pursuit, "yes-no" communication	Case-study	[23]
	Haig (1990)	1TBI	VS	6 months	100/10 mg (carbidopa) 2×/day	+	Response to command, verbal communication	Case-study	[22]
Bromocriptine	Passler (2001)	5TBI	VS	33–50 days	1.25 mg 2×/day then 2.5 mg 2×/week for 2–6 months	+	Rate of transition VS-MCS larger than normal, ↑ DRS and CRS-R scores, functional communication	Case-study	[26]
Apomorphine	Fridman (2010)	8TBI	VS/MCS	1–4 months	±5 mgmL^{-1}, begins with ratio of 2 mgh^{-1} for 12 h/day up to 8 mgh^{-1} for 12–16 h/day for 6 months	+	↑ awakening, ↑ CNC and DRS scores, response to command, functional communication for all except one patient	Case-study	[28]
	Fridman (2009)	1TBI	MCS	104 days	±5 mgmL^{-1}, begins with ratio of 2 mgh^{-1} for 12 h/day up to 8 mgh^{-1} for 12–16 h/day for 6 months	+	Response to command, "yes-no" communication, ↑ CNC, DRS, GOS scores	Prospective case-study	[27]

Methylphenidate	Martin (2007)	22 (17 TBI)	VS/MCS	3 months to 8 years	Between 7.5 and 25 mg 2×/day	/	No difference in the rate and accuracy of responses to command	Retrospective meta-analysis	[31]
	Moein (2006)	40TBI	Severe lesion	<3 weeks	Between 0.3 and 20 mg/kg/dose 2×/day during hospitalization	+	↓ duration of hospital stay (23%)	Prospective, double-blind placebo controlled randomized	[30]
Drug combinations	Patrick (2003)	10 (7 TBI)	VS/MCS	22 days to 4 months	Amantadine 100–200 mg/day, bromocriptine 0.125–400 mg/day, methylphenidate 10–80 mg/day, levodopa 25/100 mg/day or pramipexole 0.125–0.5 mg/day for 7–132 days	+	↑ WNSSP scores, ↑ responses to structured stimuli, ↑ of the recuperation ratio	Case-study, ABA paradigm	[34]
GABAergic agent									
Zolpidem	Whyte (2009)	15 (8TBI)	VS/MCS	3 months to 23 years	10 mg	+ and /	Only one responder to treatment (VS to MCS), ↑ score CRS-R, visual pursuit, response to command	Multicentric, double-blind randomized	[41]
	Cohen (2008)	1anox	MCS	8 months	5 mg/day then 10 mg/day for 3 weeks then 20 mg/day	+	↑ arousal, ↑ interactions, ↑ verbal and social responses	Case-study	[39]
	Shames (2008)	1anox	MCS	18 months	10 mg	+	↑ arousal, ↑ RLAS score, ↑ verbal communication, reading, counting, verbal production, auto-alimentation	Case-study	[40]
	Singh (2008)	1TBI	MCS	4 years	10 mg/day for 1 week	/	No effect on tests with instructions which ↑ in complexity	Single-blind case-study	[43]

(continued)

Table 12.1 (continued)

Pharmacological agent	Study (first author, year)	*N*/etiol.	Diagnostic	Interval lesion-treatment	Treatment	Effect	Results	Type of study	Ref
	Lo (2008)	2anox	VS	±1 month	10 mg for 2 days, repeated once 2 days later	/	No arousal improvement, no recovering of consciousness, no ↑ GCS score	Double-blind case-study	[42]
	Brefel-Courbon (2007)	1anox	MCS	2 years	20 mg/day for 1 week	+	↑ arousal, ↑ motor and neuropsychological performance (functional communication, eating, walking, reading and repeating words)	Prospective double-blind, placebo controlled randomized	[38]
	Clauss (2006)	2TBI and 1 anox	VS	3–5 years	10 mg/day for 3, 5 and 6 years	+	↑ arousal, ↑ GCS and RLAS scores	Case-study	[36]
	Clauss (2000)	1TBI	Semi-comatose	3 years	10 mg	+	Verbal response after 15 min, talking, answering simple questions, spontaneous interaction, counting, writing	Case-study	[35]
Baclofen	Sara (2009)	5(2TBI)	VS	6–10 months	100 mg/day continuously, up to 200 mg/day	+	↑ arousal, ↑ CRS-R score, response to command	Case-study	[51]
	Sara (2007)	1non-TBI	VS	19 months	100 mg/day continuously, up to 200 mg/day	+	VS to MCS, verbal communication, "yes-non" communication, eating, emotional response	Case-study	[49]
	Taira (2007)	2TBI	VS	1.5–2.5 months	50 mg/day for 3 day then 75 mg/day for 10 days and 100 mg/day for 10 days then 50 mg/day for 5 days then 100 mg/day for 23 days	+	↑ arousal, response to command	Case-study	[50]
	Kawecki (2007)	1TBI	VS	18 days	100 mg/day	+	Spasticity, motor and sensory aphasia improvement	Case-study	[48]

Serotoninergic agent									
Sertaline	Meythaler (2001)	11TBI	Severe lesion	<2 weeks	100 mg/day for 2 weeks	/	No improvement	Prospective, placebo controlled randomized blinded	[53]
Amitriptyline and desipramine	Reinhard (1996)	3TBI	Severe lesion	2–19 months	50–75 mg/day	+	↑ arousal and initiation, response to command, "yes-no" communication, verbal communication	Case-study	[54]
Anti-convulsive agent									
Lamotrigine	Showalter (2000)	13 (6TBI)	Severe lesion	20 days to 10 months	150–400 mg	+	↑ of consciousness and cognition, discharge from hospital sooner than expected	Case-study	[55]

N number of patients, *etiol* etiology, *TBI* traumatic brain injury, *anox* anoxia, *VS* vegetative state, *MCS* minimally conscious state, *d* day, *w* week, *mg* milligram, ↑ improvement, ↓ decrease, + positive, / no effect, *MMSE* Mini Mental State Examination, *GOS* Glasgow Outcome Scale, *DRS* Disability Rating Scale, *CRS-R* Coma Recovery Scale-Revised, *RLAS* Rancho Los Amigos Scale, *GCS* Glasgow Coma Scale, *CNC* Coma Near Coma Scale, *WNSSP* Western Neuro Sensory Program Stimulation

the results obtained. A spontaneous recovery may, however, also occur very late in patients with DOC.

Zafonte et al. reported a dose-dependent response to amantadine in a minimally conscious patient examined 5 months after a cranial trauma. During the treatment, the patient recovered his communication abilities and the score on the coma/near coma (CNC) scale [13] increased. This effect was reversible when the treatment was stopped; and during its reintroduction, the patient could communicate again [14]. Schnakers et al. have also shown the benefits of amantadine in a patient who had been in a post-anoxic minimally conscious state for 2 years and who only presented visual pursuit. Following the treatment, he was able to answer commands and the scores of the coma recovery scale-revised (CRS-R) increased [15, 16]. Amantadine has been shown to improve consciousness but also to reduce fatigue, distraction, and aggressiveness among 30 patients evaluated between 2 months and 12 years after a traumatic brain injury [17]. Finally, in a pediatric population, an improvement has been observed on behavioral scales (CNC, DRS, and Western NeuroSensory Stimulation Profile: WSSNP) [18] after taking amantadine and pramipexol (a dopamine antagonist) in ten children with severe traumatic injury [19]. On the other hand, in a group of 123 patients who suffered a severe cranial trauma, the rate of recovery of consciousness was not different between the treatment and the control group [20].

All the studies quoted up to now used only behavioral scales to objectify the effects of the amantadine treatment. Only one study by Schnakers et al. used positron emission tomography (PET) to show an increase in the cerebral metabolic activity in the frontoparietal network, which is known to be critical for the emergence of consciousness [21], and the sensitivomotor areas in a minimally conscious patient after the administration of amantadine [16].

Levodopa

As amantadine, levodopa is a dopaminergic agent initially indicated in the treatment of Parkinson's disease. A remarkable recovery has been observed in a 24-year-old man with a cranial trauma diagnosed in a vegetative state for 6 months and who was able to speak a few days after the administration of levodopa [22]. Note that no standardized validated diagnostic behavioral assessment was performed and this study like any other of the presented reports has also been published before the introduction, in 2002, of the criteria of the minimally conscious state, and thus the initial diagnosis of vegetative state might have been inaccurate. Five other DOC patients with traumatic lesions also became more responsive after taking levodopa, which was initially given to treat extrapyramidal signs [23, 24]. Finally, in a last uncontrolled unblinded study, eight vegetative patients recovered signs of consciousness after the administration of progressive amounts of levodopa. All patients could respond to commands within the firsts 2 weeks of treatment and seven of them, including two assessed more than 9 months postinjury, were able to interact in a functional way [25].

Bromocriptine

Bromocriptine is another dopamine agonist used primarily to treat Parkinson's disease. This agent, less studied, is mainly an agonist of the postsynaptic dopamine D2 receptors. It has been associated with a higher rate of patients recovering from a posttraumatic persistent vegetative state to a minimally conscious state in a retrospective study [26].

Apomorphine

Apomorphine is a nonselective dopaminergic agonist, which activates D1 and D2 receptors with a preference for the latter. This therapy was initially indicated to treat Parkinson's disease and erectile impotence but it has also shown positive effects in a few severe brain-injured patients. A minimally conscious patient treated with apomorphine 104 days after a brain trauma suddenly recovered consciousness after one day of treatment. He was able to move his legs upon request and to answer yes–no questions, which was not the case before [27]. The patient recovered full consciousness and a considerable functional recovery was maintained even after stopping the treatment. Diffusion tensor imaging showed a reduction in thalamocortical and corticothalamic projections, as expected in these patients. Another uncontrolled case-study on eight vegetative and minimally conscious patients with traumatic etiology who were treated continuously with apomorphine showed a recovery of consciousness for all patients except one, with an increase in the CNC and DRS scores [28]. These improvements lasted for at least 1 year, even after stopping the treatment.

Methylphenidate

This agent was initially used for children presenting attention deficit hyperactivity disorders and was also prescribed for narcoleptic patients. This neurostimulant increases the release of dopamine and noradrenalin while blocking the reuptake and inhibiting monoamine oxydase [29].

Few studies have been conducted and no conclusive evidence supports the use of a psycho-stimulant to improve the level of consciousness in DOC patients. Only one study suggests that the early use of methylphenidate in intensive care is associated with shorter hospital stays after severe trauma [30]. On the other hand, a recent meta-analysis on 22 chronic patients with severe brain damage (17 of traumatic etiology) did not show any clinical improvement on the percentage of responses to command after the administration of methylphenidate [31].

This pharmacological agent could rather have an effect on attention in the acute and subacute phases of recovery. Indeed, a subjective improvement of mood, of work-output, and vigilance was reported among 14 brain-traumatized patients having attention and memory deficits and being treated with methylphenidate [32]. Other studies showed similar positive effects of methylphenidate on attention and memory in patients suffering from moderate brain injury [33].

Finally, ten children and teenagers in a vegetative state and minimally conscious state were treated with a combination of dopaminergic drugs (amantadine, methylphenidate, bromocriptine, levodopa, pramipexole) and presented an improvement of responses to structured stimuli in an uncontrolled, unblinded prospective study [34].

Zolpidem

Zolpidem is an imidazopyridine which acts like an agonist on subtype 1 of the inhibiting receptors of the gamma-aminobutyric acid ($GABA_A$). This agent was initially recommended in the treatment of insomnia and presents sedative, anticonvulsive, anxiolytic, and myorelaxant effects.

A number of studies have reported the use of zolpidem as an "awakening" agent among vegetative and minimally conscious patients. This drug produces, occasionally, a clear paradoxical temporary effect on the level of consciousness in patients with severe brain damage. The effect of zolpidem has been described for the first time in 2000 after the fortuitous discovery in an allegedly vegetative patient with cranial trauma for more than 3 years and who started to speak and communicate with his family 20 min after the administration of the medication [35]. Clauss et al. reported impressive effects of this drug in four vegetative patients who had suffered a traumatic or anoxic cerebral lesion 3–5 years before [35, 36]. The patients were able to answer questions, speak, and feed themselves shortly after taking a single dose of zolpidem (10 mg). Improvements were also observed for the GCS scale (increasing from 5–9 to 10–15) and the Rancho Los Amigos scale (from III to V–VII) [37]. The level of consciousness of these patients returned to its initial state 4 h after the administration of the drug but an improvement was observed again at the time of readministration. Similar transitory effects were also reported among patients in a minimally conscious state resulting from cerebral anoxia [38–40].

Only one study investigated the percentage of responders among patients in a vegetative state and in a minimally conscious state [39]. Among 15 patients, only one indicated a significant clinical response passing from vegetative to minimally conscious state. The remaining 14 patients did not show any improvement. The rate of response to zolpidem would, thus, be close to 7%. Whyte et al. suggest that the effect of zolpidem is bimodal rather than gradual since no tendency for improvement of performance was observed among patients who did not respond to the treatment. Some case-studies also underlined the absence of improvement among patients suffering from a postanoxic encephalopathy or a severe cerebral trauma [41–43].

Several studies were interested in the mechanisms able to explain the effect of zolpidem. Single photon emission computed tomography studies showed that zolpidem increases the cerebral metabolism of hypoactive areas following traumatic or anoxic lesions [35, 36, 44]. In the same way, using PET in a minimally conscious patient, improvement of neuropsychological performances was correlated with an increase in cerebral metabolism in the frontal and postrolandic areas after taking zolpidem. Activations were also observed in anterior cingular and orbitofrontal cortex, areas known to be involved in motivational processes. A mechanism of cell dormancy was introduced to explain the effect of zolpidem: certain nonspecific areas of the brain, adjacent or distant to the initially damaged zones (e.g., the ipsilateral, contralateral hemisphere, or the cerebellum), would be inhibited by the lesion. These inactive parts of the brain would recover their function after taking zolpidem [35, 38, 44, 45], generating a recovery of consciousness. A recent study using magnetoencephalography also showed that zolpidem decreased the number of pathological slow waves associated to dormant cerebral tissue in a patient having undergone a cerebrovascular accident [46].

Zolpidem could, thus, interact with the limbic loops of the brain by modulating subcortical connections, and more particularly the globus pallidus, which would bring the thalamocortical activity back to normal and would allow a recovery of consciousness (see the mesocircuit model) [47]. From a molecular point of view, changes could take place at the level of glutamate and GABA neurotransmitters close to the cerebral lesions. The release of glutamate produces an excitotoxicity and an excess of inhibitory GABA neurotransmitters as well as a long-term oversensitiveness of the $GABA_A$ receptors [35]. The inhibitory neurotransmitters, while binding to the receptors of the ionic channels, generate a reduction of metabolism and blood flow in the adjacent cerebral areas, thus, causing a state of cells dormancy. While binding to $GABA_A$ receptors of dormant cells, zolpidem provokes the inversion of the abnormal state of the neurons and associated metabolic inhibition.

Baclofen

Baclofen is an agonist agent of the $GABA_B$ receptors, which acts on the posterior horn of the spinal cord and which is used mainly against spasticity. Spasticity, a frequent symptom following central nervous system lesions, can limit voluntary movements in patients with DOC. Baclofen, crossing with difficulty the hematoencephalic barrier, the antispasmodic effect remains modest when it is administered orally. Therefore, a direct and continuous perfusion of baclofen in low doses in the cerebrospinal fluid can be an effective treatment. Intrathecal baclofen therapy can be a useful treatment against severe spasticity among DOC patients improving the quality of life by reducing pain related spasms but also by controlling persistent autonomic dysfunctions such as tachycardia, tachypnea, fever, and breathing difficulties.

Among vegetative patients who were treated with baclofen, some impressive cases of recovery were reported in uncontrolled case-studies [48–50]. An 8-year-old boy, who sustained a severe brain injury following a car accident, received baclofen to treat his spasticity 2 months and a half after the accident. Three days after the treatment, the patient started to pronounce words, to answer verbal requests, and subsequently showed good recovery. Similarly, an 18-year-old man diagnosed in a vegetative state received intrathecal baclofen 1 month and a half after his brain trauma. Five days later, he was able to answer verbal requests and he subsequently recovered motor and cognitive capacities [50]. Another case-study also showed an impressive recovery in an 11-year-old girl presenting a vegetative state on admission due to diffuse axonal injury following a car accident. After 18 days, she was treated with intrathecal baclofen and she recovered from spasticity, motor, and sensory aphasia [48]. Note, however, that the time postinsult was relatively short in these three patients and spontaneous recovery might have occurred as well.

A positive effect of baclofen was also observed in five allegedly vegetative patients treated for spasticity in the chronic stage (at least 19 months after the injury). Two weeks after, all except one patient presented clinical improvement, which remained stable until the end of the 6-months follow-up. Improvements went from a high increase in vigilance to a recovery of consciousness, as revealed by the changes in the CRS-R scores [51]. Finally, in one last case-study, following the introduction of intrathecal baclofen, a 44-year-old man recovered consciousness 19 months after a nontraumatic brain injury (i.e., subarachnoid hemorrhage due to a ruptured aneurysm). He however remains dependent on others for his daily activities [49].

Several assumptions have been made to explain the effects of baclofen on recovery of consciousness. Some authors suggest a modulation of motor impulses of the spinal cord on the possible cortical reactivation [51]. Baclofen would improve nervous conduction in the demyelinized axons and could possibly accelerate the restoration of diffuse axonal injury [52]. A modulation of the sleep–wake cycle has also been considered as a mechanism responsible for the effect of baclofen [51]. But all these explanations at present remain hypothetical.

Serotonin-Reuptake Inhibitors

Sertalin is an antidepressant of the selective serotonin reuptake inhibitor class. Acute brain lesions have been reported to increase cerebral serotonin but in the chronic phase a downregulation of the serotonin system is thought to occur. In a prospective placebo-controlled randomized study, sertalin treatment did not improve the level of consciousness among 11 severely brain-injured patients [53]. On the other hand, amitriptylin and desipramin treatment (tricyclic antidepressants also blocking the recapture of serotonin) improved recovery in three patients with severe traumatic brain injury in an uncontrolled unblinded study [54]. Two of these patients presented deterioration when the drug was stopped, but an improvement was again observed at the time of reintroduction of the treatment. The third patient started to talk after being mute for more than 1 year. The possible mechanisms of action in this context remain largely unexplained.

Lamotrigin

Lamotrigin is an antiepileptic agent used in the treatment of epilepsy and bipolar disorders. By inhibiting the voltage-dependent sodium channels, it stabilizes the neuronal membrane and inhibits glutamate release, an excitatory neurotransmitter. The effects on the sodium ion channels contribute to the antiepileptic effects while the antiglutamatergic agents act more on the psychotropic effects with a possible neuroprotective action. Functional improvement of DOC patients has been observed after administration of lamotrigin, showing recovery of consciousness and cognition combined with an earlier discharge from hospital [55]. This uncontrolled unblinded study concluded a possible effect on functional recovery, and particularly in patients who had already emerged from the minimally conscious state.

Mechanisms Aiming to Explain the Possible Positive Effects of Pharmacological Treatments

Each drug affects one or more neuronal pathways. Amantadine, levodopa, bromocriptine, methylphenidate, and apomorphine act mainly on the dopaminergic system; whereas, zolpidem and baclofen affect preferentially the gabaergic system (albeit at different locations in the nervous system), while sertraline, amitriptyline, and desipramine interfere rather in serotoninergic processes. The subjacent neurological mechanisms to the positive effects of these drugs are currently not well-understood. As we have seen, amantadine and zolpidem would increase the metabolism of hypoactive cerebral regions [16, 56]. Zolpidem would play a main role in the gabaergic system of the limbic loops in the brain [57]; whereas, baclofen would act more on the spinal cord and would support the regeneration of motor neurons [51].

The *model of the mesocircuit* has been proposed recently to explain the various pharmacological effects on the recovery of consciousness [47, 57] (Fig. 12.1). The central thalamic nuclei (CTN) seem particularly important in the emergence of consciousness. They receive ascending projections coming from the brainstem encompassing the arousal systems that control the activity of many cortical and thalamic neurons during the sleep–wake cycle. The CTN are strongly nerved by cholinergic, serotoninergic, noradrenergic afferents of the arousal systems in the brainstem.

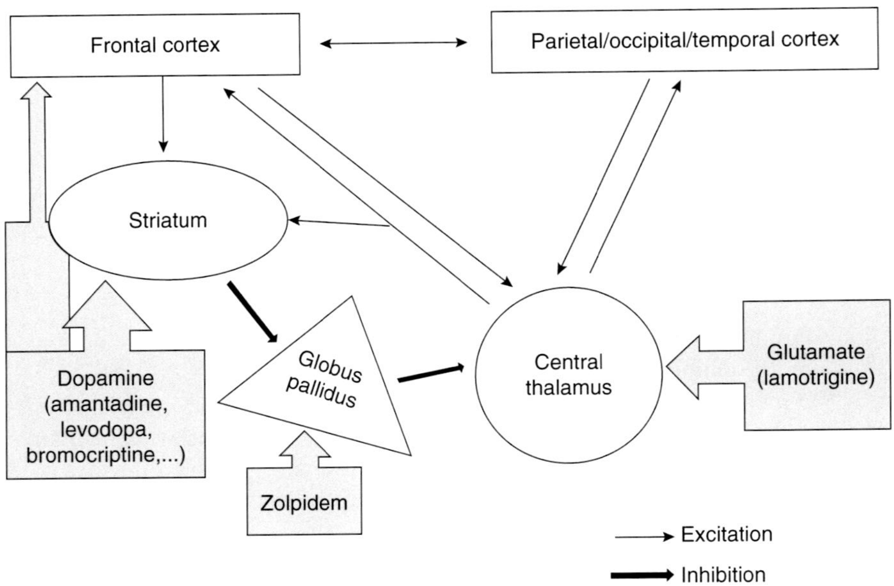

Fig. 12.1 Model of the mesocircuit that aims to explain the mechanisms of pharmacologically induced recovery of consciousness (Adapted from [47])

These same neurons of the CTN are also innervated by the downward projections coming from the areas of the frontoparietal cortex. Collectively, these ascending and descending pathways seem to modulate the level of consciousness [57]. The frontoparietal cortex (and its subcortical modulation via striatum, globus pallidus, and thalamus) is also prevalent for the emergence of consciousness. Thalamocortical projections coming from the CTN activate in normal conditions the neurons of the cortex and striatum. Lesions at this level result in a reduction of cerebral metabolism. Neurons of the striatum inhibit the internal globus pallidus but require a strong basic synaptic activity and elevated levels of dopaminergic innervations in order to maintain their state in activity. Without projections of the striatum to the globus pallidus (e.g., by a lack of dopaminergic innervations), the globus pallidus itself will inhibit the CTN, which in turn will inhibit the cortical structures, and this sequence could, thus, generate consciousness disorders. Disturbances in this mesocircuit influence the total dynamics of the dominating corticothalamic and frontoparietal systems [58]. Dopaminergic drugs could, therefore, facilitate projections of the striatum on the globus pallidus, which would modulate the frontoparietal cortical neurons and would restore the corticosubcortical loops. Zolpidem is thought to act directly on the globus pallidus and would make it possible to inhibit it (as it is usually the case due to the action of the striatum), which would also restore the activity of the CTN, whereas the glutamatergic agents (e.g., lamotrigine) would intervene directly on the CTN (Fig. 12.1).

Conclusion

No strong evidence currently supports or disproves the specific use of a pharmacological agent in order to improve the level of consciousness in DOC patients. As discussed, a number of small and uncontrolled case or cohort studies have reported a positive clinical response. Indeed, transitory or permanent improvements were observed among some vegetative or minimally conscious patients of various etiologies (traumatic brain injury, cerebrovascular accident, anoxia, etc.). Reported effects were variable, ranging from increase in wakefulness, partial recovery of consciousness, motor, verbal, or communication functions to full recovery of cognitive functioning.

Some of the reviewed treatments seem to benefit patients with severe disorders of consciousness (e.g., amantadine, zolpidem, baclofen), whereas others (e.g., methylphenidate, lamotrigine) seem to possibly be more beneficial for brain-damaged but conscious patients improving their attention deficit disorder [59]. The effects were observed in the short- and long-term, and this, generated by a single dose (e.g., zolpidem) or by a continuous treatment (e.g., amantadine, baclofen, levodopa).

To date, the absence of double-blind placebo-controlled randomized multicentric studies does not permit to propose any evidence-based therapeutic guidelines for a specific diagnostic entity of DOC (vegetative versus minimally conscious state), taking into account etiology and duration of the brain damage. Indeed, the reported data come from case or cohort reports presenting methodological limitations and not permitting to disentangle the drug effect from the natural evolution of the disease. Studies including a broader number of patients are especially influenced by the extreme heterogeneity of DOC, such as the site of neuropathological lesions, time elapsed between injury and the introduction of the treatment, confounding drugs received, and medical comorbidities. Moreover, it is difficult to compare between studies since they lack homogeneity in methodology and differ in the duration of treatment, administered doses, and patients' demographics and clinical status (Table 12.1). Measurement tools and behavioral scales are also very different across studies (e.g., CRS-R, DRS, GCS, CNC, WSSNP) and a standardization of bedside assessment seems necessary. The most adapted scale in this context is the coma recovery scale-revised which has been specifically developed to distinguish between vegetative and minimally conscious patients [60]. Obviously, placebo-controlled, double-blind randomized multicentric studies are necessary before drawing any conclusion on the effectiveness of therapeutic treatments in these challenging patients.

Even if several hypotheses have been proposed, such as the mesocircuit model, there is still a need to better understand the mechanisms and involved neurotransmitters systems underlying residual neural plasticity and recovery from severe brain damage. It would also be necessary to develop biomarkers of consciousness recovery using neuroimagery or electrophysiology and to better define therapeutic responders (e.g., genetic markers). It could also be useful (albeit methodologically more complicated) to test the efficacy of a combination of different pharmatherapeutic agents and/or combinations with nonpharmacological rehabilitation interventions and this by refining the timing of coercive interventions (therapy based on amount and intensity). The nonpharmacological interventions such as physical and cognitive rehabilitation as well as the sensory stimulation programs are complementary and essential in the therapy planning of DOC patients. Finally, deep brain stimulation is currently being investigated as a therapeutic option in some selected patients with posttraumatic minimally conscious state but still remains in the research field and should be more investigated before being implemented in the clinical routine [61].

References

1. Brown EN, Lydic R, Schiff ND. General anesthesia, sleep and coma. N Engl J Med. 2010;363(27):2638–50.
2. The Multi-Society Task Force on PVS. Medical aspects of the persistent vegetative state (1). N Engl J Med. 1994;330(21):1499–508.
3. Giacino JT, Ashwal S, Childs N, et al. The minimally conscious state: definition and diagnostic criteria. Neurology. 2002;58(3):349–53.
4. Bruno MA, Vanhaudenhuyse A, Thibaut A, Moonen G, Laureys S. From unresponsive wakefulness to minimally conscious PLUS and functional locked-in syndromes: recent advances in our understanding of disorders of consciousness. J Neurol. 2011;258(7):1373–84.
5. Lombardi F, Taricco M, De Tanti A, Telaro E, Liberati A. Sensory stimulation of brain-injured individuals in coma or vegetative state: results of a Cochrane systematic review, Clin Rehabil. 2002;16(5):464–72.
6. Zafonte R, Lexell J, Cullen N. Possible applications for dopaminergic agents following traumatic brain injury: part 2. J Head Trauma Rehabil. 2001;16(1):112–6.
7. Born JD. The Glasgow-Liège Scale. Prognostic value and evaluation of motor response and brain stem reflexes after severe head injury. Acta Neurochir. 1988;95:49–52.
8. Saniova B, Drobny M, Kneslova L, et al. The outcome of patients with severe head injuries treated with amantadine sulphate. J Neural Transm. 2004;111(4):511–4.
9. Folstein M, Robins L, Helzer J. The mini-mental state examination. Arch Gen Psychiatry. 1983;40(7):812.
10. Jennett B, Bond M. Assessment of outcome after severe brain damage. Lancet. 1975; 1(7905):480–4.
11. Rappaport M, Hall KM, Hopkins K, et al. Disability rating scale for severe head trauma: coma to community. Arch Phys Med Rehabil. 1982;63(3):118–23.
12. Meythaler JM, Brunner RC, Johnson A, et al. Amantadine to improve neurorecovery in traumatic brain injury-associated diffuse axonal injury: a pilot double-blind randomized trial. J Head Trauma Rehabil. 2002;17(4):300–13.
13. Rappaport M. The coma/near coma scale. 2000. Retrieved 21 Aug 21, 2006, from http://www.tbims.org/combi/cnc
14. Zafonte R, Watanabe T, Mann N. Amantadine: a potential treatment for the minimally conscious state. Brain Inj. 1998;12(7):617–21.
15. Giacino JT, Kalmar K, Whyte J. The JFK Coma Recovery Scale-Revised: measurement characteristics and diagnostic utility. Arch Phys Med Rehabil. 2004;85(12):2020–9.
16. Schnakers C, Hustinx R, Vandewalle G, et al. Measuring the effect of amantadine in chronic anoxic minimally conscious state. J Neurol Neurosurg Psychiatry. 2008;79(2):225–7.
17. Gualtieri T, Chandler M, Coons T, et al. Amantadine: a new clinical profile for traumatic brain injury. Clin Neuropharmacol. 1989;12(4):258–70.

18. Ansell BJ, Keenan JE. The Western Neuro Sensory Stimulation Profile: a tool for assessing slow-to-recover head-injured patients. Arch Phys Med Rehabil. 1989;70(2):104–8.
19. Patrick P, Blackman J, Mabry J, et al. Dopamine agonist therapy in low-response children following traumatic brain injury. J Child Neurol. 2006;21(10):879–85.
20. Hughes S, Colantonio A, Santaguida P, et al. Amantadine to enhance readiness for rehabilitation following severe traumatic brain injury. Brain Inj. 2005;19(14):1197–206.
21. Laureys S, Piret S, Ledoux D. Quantifying consciousness. Lancet Neurol. 2005;4(12): 789–90.
22. Haig A, Ruess J. Recovery from vegetative state of six months' duration associated with Sinemet (levodopa/carbidopa). Arch Phys Med Rehabil. 1990;71(13):1081–3.
23. Matsuda W, Matsumura A, Komatsu Y, et al. Awakenings from persistent vegetative state: report of three cases with parkinsonism and brain stem lesions on MRI. J Neurol Neurosurg Psychiatry. 2003;74(11):1571–3.
24. Matsuda W, Komatsu Y, Yanaka K, et al. Levodopa treatment for patients in persistent vegetative or minimally conscious states. Neuropsychol Rehabil. 2005;15(3–4):414–27.
25. Krimchansky B, Keren O, Sazbon L, et al. Differential time and related appearance of signs, indicating improvement in the state of consciousness in vegetative state traumatic brain injury (VS-TBI) patients after initiation of dopamine treatment. Brain Inj. 2004;18(11):1099–105.
26. Passler MA, Riggs RV. Positive outcomes in traumatic brain injury-vegetative state: patients treated with bromocriptine. Arch Phys Med Rehabil. 2001;82(3):311–5.
27. Fridman E, Calvar J, Bonetto M, et al. Fast awakening from minimally conscious state with apomorphine. Brain Inj. 2009;23(2):172–7.
28. Fridman E, Krimchansky B, Bonetto M, et al. Continuous subcutaneous apomorphine for severe disorders of consciousness after traumatic brain injury. Brain Inj. 2010;24(4):636–41.
29. Chew E, Zafonte R. Pharmacological management of neurobehavioral disorders following traumatic brain injury–a state-of-the-art review. J Rehabil Res Dev. 2009;46(6):851–79.
30. Moein H, Khalili H, Keramatian K. Effect of methylphenidate on ICU and hospital length of stay in patients with severe and moderate traumatic brain injury. Clin Neurol Neurosurg. 2006;108(6):539–42.
31. Martin R, Whyte J. The effects of methylphenidate on command following and yes/no communication in persons with severe disorders of consciousness: a meta-analysis of n-of-1 studies. Am J Phys Med Rehabil. 2007;86(8):613–20.
32. Gualtieri C, Evans R. Stimulant treatment for the neurobehavioural sequelae of traumatic brain injury. Brain Inj. 1988;2(4):273–90.
33. Whyte J, Hart T, Vaccaro M, et al. Effects of methylphenidate on attention deficits after traumatic brain injury: a multidimensional, randomized, controlled trial. Am J Phys Med Rehabil. 2004;83(6):401–20.
34. Patrick P, Buck M, Conaway M, et al. The use of dopamine enhancing medications with children in low response states following brain injury. Brain Inj. 2003;17(6):497–506.
35. Clauss RP, Guldenpfennig WM, Nel HW, et al. Extraordinary arousal from semi-comatose state on zolpidem. A case report. S Afr Med J. 2000;90(1):68–72.
36. Clauss R, Nel W. Drug induced arousal from the permanent vegetative state. NeuroRehabilitation. 2006;21(1):23–8.
37. Hagen C, Malkmus D, Durham P. Levels of cognitive functioning. Downey: Rancho Los Amigos Hospital Inc.; 1987.
38. Brefel-Courbon C, Payoux P, Ory F, et al. Clinical and imaging evidence of zolpidem effect in hypoxic encephalopathy. Ann Neurol. 2007;62(1):102–5.
39. Cohen SI, Duong TT. Increased arousal in a patient with anoxic brain injury after administration of zolpidem. Am J Phys Med Rehabil. 2008;87(3):229–31.
40. Shames JL, Ring H. Transient reversal of anoxic brain injury-related minimally conscious state after zolpidem administration: a case report. Arch Phys Med Rehabil. 2008;89(2):386–8.
41. Whyte J, Myers R. Incidence of clinically significant responses to zolpidem among patients with disorders of consciousness: a preliminary placebo controlled trial. Am J Phys Med Rehabil. 2009;88(5):410–8.

42. Lo Y, Tan E, Ratnagopal P, et al. Zolpidem and its effects on hypoxic encephalopathy. Ann Neurol. 2008;64(4):477–8.
43. Singh R, McDonald C, Dawson K, et al. Zolpidem in a minimally conscious state. Brain Inj. 2008;22(1):103–6.
44. Cohen L, Chaaban B, Habert MO. Transient improvement of aphasia with zolpidem. N Engl J Med. 2004;350(9):949–50.
45. Clauss RP, Nel WH. Effect of zolpidem on brain injury and diaschisis as detected by 99mTc HMPAO brain SPECT in humans. Arzneimittelforschung. 2004;54(10):641–6.
46. Hall S, Yamawaki N, Fisher A, et al. GABA(A) alpha-1 subunit mediated desynchronization of elevated low frequency oscillations alleviates specific dysfunction in stroke–a case report. Clin Neurophysiol. 2010;121(4):549–55.
47. Schiff N. Recovery of consciousness after brain injury: a mesocircuit hypothesis. Trends Neurosci. 2010;33(1):1–9.
48. Kawecki Z, Kwiatkowski S, Grzegorzewski P, et al. Sudden improvement of all neurological functions after general anesthesia and two-day intrathecal infusion of baclofen in a child with primary brain-stem injury. Przegl Lek. 2007;64(2):13–4.
49. Sarà M, Sacco S, Cipolla F, et al. An unexpected recovery from permanent vegetative state. Brain Inj. 2007;21(1):101–3.
50. Taira T, Hori T. Intrathecal baclofen in the treatment of post-stroke central pain, dystonia, and persistent vegetative state. Acta Neurochir Suppl. 2007;97(Pt 1):227–9.
51. Sarà M, Pistoia F, Mura E, et al. Intrathecal baclofen in patients with persistent vegetative state: 2 hypotheses. Arch Phys Med Rehabil. 2009;90(7):1245–9.
52. Taira T. Intrathecal administration of GABA agonists in the vegetative state. Prog Brain Res. 2009;177:317–28.
53. Meythaler J, Depalma L, Devivo M, et al. Sertraline to improve arousal and alertness in severe traumatic brain injury secondary to motor vehicle crashes. Brain Inj. 2001;15(4):321–31.
54. Reinhard D, Whyte J, Sandel M. Improved arousal and initiation following tricyclic antidepressant use in severe brain injury. Arch Phys Med Rehabil. 1996;77(1):80–3.
55. Showalter P, Kimmel D. Stimulating consciousness and cognition following severe brain injury: a new potential clinical use for lamotrigine. Brain Inj. 2000;14:997–1001.
56. Clauss R. Neurotransmitters in coma, vegetative and minimally conscious states, pharmacological interventions. Med Hypotheses. 2010;75(3):287–90.
57. Schiff N. Recovery of consciousness after severe brain injury: the role of arousal regulation mechanisms and some speculation on the heart-brain interface. Cleve Clin J Med. 2010;77 Suppl 3:S27–33.
58. Laureys S, Schiff N. Coma and consciousness: paradigms (re)framed by neuroimaging. Neuroimage. 2011 Dec 27. [Epub ahead of print]
59. Pistoia F, Mura E, Govoni S, et al. Awakenings and awareness recovery in disorders of consciousness: is there a role for drugs? CNS Drugs. 2010;24(8):625–38.
60. American Congress of Rehabilitation Medicine, Brain Injury-Interdisciplinary Special Interest Group, Disorders of Consciousness Task Force, Seel R, Sherer M, Whyte J, Katz D, Giacino J, Rosenbaum A, Hammond F, Kalmar K, Pape T, Zafonte R, Biester R, Kaelin D, Kean J, Zasler N. Assessment scales for disorders of consciousness: evidence-based recommendations for clinical practice and research. Arch Phys Med Rehabil. 2010;91(12):1795–813.
61. Schiff ND, Giacino JT, Kalmar K, et al. Behavioural improvements with thalamic stimulation after severe traumatic brain injury. Nature. 2007;448(7153):600–3.

Chapter 13
Deep Brain Stimulation

Marie Thonnard

Introduction

Chronic vegetative state/unresponsive wakefulness and minimally conscious state are disorders of consciousness (DOC) that can follow severe brain lesions [1]. These states are currently relatively well-defined but their therapeutic options remain relatively limited. Reports on patients having received noninvasive (generally pharmacological) treatment are mainly uncontrolled. Often these are case reports and the methodology is frequently suboptimal to provide empirical evidences for the treatment efficiency. However, while invasive, one therapeutic technique is increasingly studied: deep brain stimulation (DBS). This technique is used as a treatment in different neurological diseases but particularly in Parkinson's disease, for which technological advances have allowed the treatment of a large number of patients. Thanks to these advances, studies related to DBS as a treatment for DOC could be developed. Even though methodological difficulties are evident, results are promising. We propose in this chapter a description of the DBS technique, an outline of previous clinical applications, review of studies using this technique in DOC patients along with a summary of mechanisms explaining the efficacy of DBS for treating these patients.

M. Thonnard, M.Sc.
Coma Science Group, Cyclotron Research Center, University of Liège,
Allée du 6 août, 8, Sart-Tilman B30, 4000 Liège, Belgium

Department of Neurology, University Hospital of Liège,
Liège, Belgium
e-mail: marie.thonnard@ulg.ac.be

C. Schnakers, S. Laureys (eds.), *Coma and Disorders of Consciousness*,
DOI 10.1007/978-1-4471-2440-5_13, © Springer-Verlag London 2012

History and Clinical Applications

DBS is a treatment aiming to stimulate target brain structures of one or both hemisphere using surgically implanted electrodes and an electrical pulse generator, also called "*brain pacemaker*" or "*neurostimulator*." Bartholow [2] was the first to report the use of this technique in humans. DBS was first used in order to localize and map functions of particular cerebral regions [3], and, later, to investigate the effects of stimulation on deep brain structures [4]. In the 1960s emerged the idea that it is possible to treat neurological disease with this technique, but it was only in the 1970s that the first trials using DBS were reported, particularly in patients with chronic pain [5], epilepsy [6], or movement disorders [7]. Thanks to technological advances of neurostimulators that can be surgically implanted, first trials about the long-term use of DBS were reported in the 1990s [8, 9]. Since then, this technique has been used to treat several neurological and psychiatric disorders such as motor disorders (e.g., essential tremor, dystonia, Parkinson's disease), Tourette's syndrome, chronic pain, or obsessive-compulsive disorders.

Nowadays, DBS is used in the treatment of several pathologies. Notably, the stimulation of ventral intermediate nucleus of the thalamus seems to be efficient in the treatment of essential tremor [9–12]. Concerning the treatment of dystonia, the stimulation of the globus pallidus and of the thalamus has shown some efficiency [13–15]. Several target brain areas are used for the treatment of Parkinson's disease, with diverse effects according to the target regions stimulated. Whereas the stimulation of the ventral intermediate nucleus significantly reduces tremor [16, 17], the stimulation of the subthalamic nucleus and of the globus pallidus also provokes a decrease of bradykinesia and hypertonia [18–22].

DBS and DOC Treatment

Previous Studies

In the literature, there are few studies on DBS in patients with DOC. Although some methodological bias could be discussed, studies performed in this area have allowed a better understanding of DBS mechanisms in DOC. Early animal studies by Moruzzi and Magoun [23] have shown that the stimulation of the midbrain reticular formation leads to electroencephalogram desynchronizations, similar to those observed in wakefulness states. Later, other studies have shown the relation between the midbrain reticular formation and the level of vigilance in both animals [24] and humans [25]. The first DBS studies in vegetative patients focused on the reticular formation, the basal ganglia, and especially, on the thalamus. Sturm et al. [26], Hassler et al. [27], and McLardy et al. [28] were the first to report clinical results using DBS in intralaminar and rostral-ventral thalamic nuclei in unconscious patients. However, their clinical results and the long-term follow-up were incomplete and suboptimal. In the 1980s, Medtronic Inc. (Minneapolis, Minnesota, USA) initiated a multicentric study involving French, Japanese, and American teams. Cohadon [29] have studied the effect of DBS on parafascicular intralaminar and centromedian thalamic nuclei in 25 patients who were in a vegetative state since at least 3 months. In this cohort, 12 patients showed no clinical or behavioral improvements in a follow-up period of 1–12 years. The remaining 13 patients manifested a significant improvement of the level of consciousness and of interpersonal interactions after 1–3 weeks of treatment. In a study by Tsubokawa et al. [30], the authors have stimulated the midbrain reticular formation (cuneiform nucleus) and unspecific thalamic nuclei (median-parafascicular complex) in eight vegetative patients (2–3 months post injury). Patients were assessed with behavioral and electrophysiological measures (e.g., electroencephalogram, brainstem auditory evoked potentials, and somatosensory evoked potentials) and behavioral improvements were reported in three cases (i.e., response to command and vocalizations/verbalizations) with a partial improvement noticed in a fourth patient (i.e., recovery of oral feeding and emotional expressions). The remaining four patients did not show any improvement after 1 year of DBS. However, even though some changes have been observed directly after the activation of the DBS device (e.g., more frequent eye and mouth opening), most behavioral improvements were recorded only after 3–4 months of treatment.

Other studies by Katayama et al. [31] and Hosobuchi and Yingling [32] have shown similar improvements in vegetative patients. However, in both studies, the observed improvements could also be explained, entirely or partially, by spontaneous recovery. Indeed, the reported improvements appeared within a 1 year postinjury period, during which a spontaneous recovery is most likely to appear. In addition, the authors did not use a placebo-controlled double-blind design or a period of DBS stimulation withdrawal. Finally, criteria of minimally conscious state having been defined only a few years ago [33], some patients could have met, a posteriori, the criteria of MCS.

Yamamoto et al. [34] have studied the effect of DBS in stimulating the midbrain reticular formation and the median-parafascicular complex of the thalamus in 21 vegetative patients and 5 minimally conscious patients. Eight vegetative patients were reported to have emerged and were able to respond to simple commands. Four out of five minimally conscious patients also had emerged (showing recovery of functional communication) and could return living at home.

Most often, results in truly "vegetative" patients did not allow to unequivocally concluding on the efficiency of DBS. In part, this could be explained by the massive brain lesions presented by vegetative patients. Indeed, in nontraumatic etiology, diffuse ischemic damages of the neocortex and severe thalamic injuries are classically encountered. In posttraumatic patients, diffuse axonal injury as well as thalamic lesions are frequently observed. In both etiologies, subcortical lesions of white matter with thalamic deafferentations can be found. Brain structures with possible residual function may not be able to function because of corticocortical and thalamocortical disconnections [35]. Thus, even though DBS of the thalamus in vegetative patients are aimed to enhance the level of wakefulness and consciousness by activating respective neuronal networks, it would be efficient only in rare cases. Indeed, DBS cannot have a significant effect on a widespread network via the thalamus if the connections within this network or between the thalamus and this network are disrupted. For traumatic lesions, often involving multifocal lesions (and thus the preservation of a larger set of neuronal connections), DBS could be more efficient. In 2007, Schiff et al. [36] have reported the case of a chronic posttraumatic patient treated with DBS of thalamic intralaminar nuclei in a double-blind design with recording of several baselines. Clinically, the patient was in a minimally conscious state and was 6 years postinjury, decreasing the possibility of a spontaneous recovery. In addition, the patient did not show any improvement despite several previous rehabilitation programs. Behavioral changes were assessed with the coma recovery scale-revised [37] and with objects denomination, motor limb control, and oral feeding tests. Improvements appeared after the placement of the *neurostimulator*. Intelligible verbalizations and functional object use were already reported during the titration phase. Later, responses to command, spontaneous limb movements, oral feeding, and, especially, a recovery of functional communication were observed.

The methodology of this last case report seems to compensate the bias observed in previous studies. Indeed, the authors have used several baselines to be sure that the observed changes were linked to the presence of the treatment and could not be attributed to the ongoing rehabilitation program. Besides, for such a chronic patient, the probability of changes due to a spontaneous recovery was very small (but not inexistent) [38]. Importantly, brain imaging in this patient showed neither lesions in language-related regions nor lesions in the thalamus.

Mechanisms Involved in DOC Treatment Using DBS

Consciousness seems to be underlined by a large network of cortical regions (e.g., frontoparietal) but also by thalamo-cortical and cortico-cortical connectivity [39, 40]. Damages within this network can lead to DOC. Indeed, in the minimally conscious state, this network would be more preserved than in the vegetative state. The thalamus plays an important role in consciousness processing as it has many connections with this fronto-parietal "awareness-network". Hence, a thalamic lesion can be responsible for severe DOC. The aim of stimulating the thalamus would be to reactivate connections within this network in compensating for the lack of thalamic activation. Thereby, DBS of the thalamus would have a higher efficacy in patients with a relatively preserved thalamocortical axonal network.

Within the thalamus, intralaminar nuclei seem to be particularly connected with higher level cortical areas. Previous studies have shown selective vulnerability of neurons within central nuclei of the thalamus. Indeed, cellular loss in these particular nuclei would be strongly associated with the patients' level of recovery [35, 41]. Whereas the level of functioning is higher in patients with lesions of anterior and median central nuclei, an additional damage in intralaminar regions often results in a severe inability or even a vegetative state. The central nuclei of the thalamus, and particularly the intralaminar nuclei, seem therefore to play a central role in DOC pathology. The central nuclei seem to play a key-role in wakefulness and vigilance functions as regards their high number of connections with the brainstem and the basal midbrain [42]. In addition, activity in central nuclei of the thalamus could vary according to the level of vigilance and according to the cognitive workload required to achieve a task [25], explaining performance fluctuations usually observed in DOC.

Intralaminar Nuclei of the Thalamus as a Target for DBS

In the treatment of DOC, the target area for DBS that would offer the best results seems to be the intralaminar nuclei of the thalamus and this for several reasons [43]. First, the central thalamus is supposed to be altered as regards pathophysiological mechanisms linked to traumatic brain injury, which are diffuse axonal damage, downward displacement of the thalamus and the brainstem; and/or ischemic lesions of the brainstem, the midbrain, the thalamus, and of the basal ganglia. Indeed, diffuse axonal lesions lead to axonal disconnections within a large brain network, generating an extensive neuronal death. As mentioned earlier, cellular loss in central thalamus seems to be particularly associated with DOC patients' level of recovery [35, 41]. Then, a traumatic brain injury generally leads to a decrease in forebrain activity and that partly because of the role of central thalamic nuclei. As mentioned earlier, central thalamic neurons are important in attention and wakefulness regulations. These neurons could be monitored by the wakefulness level generated by ascending brainstem connections [44], but also by medial frontal regions that calibrate the level of cortical activation during cognitive tasks [25]. Thereby, lesions of these regions could decrease the activity in the ipsilateral hemisphere and cause bilateral metabolic dysfunctions. Finally, DBS seems to generate action potentials in intact axonal fibers. Central and intralaminar nuclei neurons release an excitatory neurotransmitter, glutamate, which provokes a depolarization of striatum and cortex. When the striatum is activated, this can produce a large pattern of brain activations. Thus, in compensating for neuronal activity in the central thalamus, the stimulation of these neurons using DBS could facilitate the induction and maintaining the activity in a large network of neurons through the entire brain and thus lead to the recovery of cognitive functions underlined by these networks (e.g., attention, memory, language, executive functions, etc.). Finally, a sustained DBS of intralaminar thalamic nuclei could have long-term behavioral effects, such as those observed in the study of Schiff et al. [36]. Indeed, in this patient initially diagnosed as being in a minimally conscious state, improvements persisted during the stimulation withdrawal period. Similar changes have also been reported in animals treated with repetitive DBS. These long-term effects could reflect neuroplasticity phenomena that await further characterization and understanding.

Conclusion

The controlled study of DBS as a potential treatment for DOC is relatively recent. Evolving in parallel to technological advances and scientific discoveries, studies about DBS in DOC tend to show promising results. However, older studies present methodological bias considering present knowledge, particularly as regards patients' selection, target area for DBS and methodological design. Previous studies have nevertheless allowed highlighting several criteria for the DBS use in DOC patients: (1) selection of posttraumatic patients, nontraumatic lesions generally affecting a larger number of brain regions and connections; (2) selection of patients at least 1 year post injury, in order to decrease the effect of spontaneous recovery; (3) selection of patients in a minimally conscious state, vegetative patients usually showing widespread axonal injury and larger brain disconnections; (4) selection of patients showing no lesions in the thalamus or in regions crucial to consciousness recovery (e.g., frontoparietal and language regions); (5) the use of a valid experimental design (e.g., double-blind and baseline measurements); (6) a rehabilitation program maintained and unchanged during the DBS trial, in order to verify that improvements are due to stimulation and not to the rehabilitation program. The study by Schiff et al. [36] has notably allowed showing DBS-related improvements taking into account all recommendations aforementioned. Nevertheless, it remains a case report that does not allow generalizing results to a larger population of patients. Therefore, the application of such an invasive methodology in a bigger sample is necessary to validate the DBS use as a treatment for DOC, taking into account the challenging ethical issues involved [45].

References

1. Laureys S, Owen AM, Schiff ND. Brain function in coma, vegetative state, and related disorders. Lancet Neurol. 2004;3:537–46.
2. Bartholow R. Experimental investigations into the functions of the human brain. Am J Med Sci. 1874;67:305–16.
3. Penfield W, Boldrey E. Somatic motor and sensory representation in the cerebral cortex of man as studied by electrical stimulation. Brain. 1937;60:389–443.
4. Spiegel EA, Wycis HT, Marks M, Lee AJ. Stereotaxic apparatus for operations on the human brain. Science. 1947;106:349–50.
5. Hosobuchi Y, Adams JE, Rutkin B. Chronic thalamic stimulation for the control of facial anesthesia dolorosa. Arch Neurol. 1973;29:158–61.
6. Cooper IS. Effect of chronic stimulation of anterior cerebellum on neurological disease. Lancet. 1973;1:206.
7. Brice J, McLellan L. Suppression of intention tremor by contingent deep-brain stimulation. Lancet. 1980;1:1221.
8. Benabid AL, Pollak P, Gervason C, et al. Long-term suppression of tremor by chronic stimulation of the ventral intermediate thalamic nucleus. Lancet. 1991;337:403–6.
9. Benabid AL, Pollak P, Gao D, et al. Chronic electrical stimulation of the ventralis intermedius nucleus of the thalamus as a treatment of movement disorders. J Neurosurg. 1996;84:203–14.

10. Koller WC, Lyons KE, Wilkinson SB, Pahwa R. Efficacy of unilateral deep brain stimulation of the VIM nucleus of the thalamus for essential head tremor. Mov Disord. 1999;14:847–50.
11. Ondo W, Jankovic J, Schwartz K, et al. Unilateral thalamic deep brain stimulation for refractory essential tremor and Parkinson's disease tremor. Neurology. 1998;51:1063–9.
12. Rehncrona S, Johnels B, Widner H, et al. Long-term efficacy of thalamic deep brain stimulation for tremor: double-blind assessments. Mov Disord. 2003;18:163–70.
13. Kumar R, Dagher A, Hutchison WD, et al. Globus pallidus deep brain stimulation for generalized dystonia: clinical and PET investigation. Neurology. 1999;53:871–4.
14. Sellal F, Hirsch E, Barth P, et al. A case of symptomatic hemidystonia improved by ventroposterolateral thalamic electrostimulation. Mov Disord. 1993;8:515–8.
15. Lozano AM, Kumar R, Gross RE, et al. Globus pallidus internus pallidotomy for generalized dystonia. Mov Disord. 1997;12:865–70.
16. Kumar R, Lozano AM, Sime E, Lang AE. Long-term follow-up of thalamic deep brain stimulation for essential and parkinsonian tremor. Neurology. 2003;61:1601–4.
17. Putzke JD, Wharen Jr RE, Wszolek ZK, et al. Thalamic deep brain stimulation for tremor-predominant Parkinson's disease. Parkinsonism Relat Disord. 2003;10:81–8.
18. Anderson VC, Burchiel KJ, Hogarth P, et al. Pallidal vs subthalamic nucleus deep brain stimulation in Parkinson disease. Arch Neurol. 2005;62:554–60.
19. Peppe A, Pierantozzi M, Altibrandi MG, et al. Bilateral GPi DBS is useful to reduce abnormal involuntary movements in advanced Parkinson's disease patients, but its action is related to modality and site of stimulation. Eur J Neurol. 2001;8:579–86.
20. Loher TJ, Burgunder JM, Weber S, et al. Effect of chronic pallidal deep brain stimulation on off period dystonia and sensory symptoms in advanced Parkinson's disease. J Neurol Neurosurg Psychiatry. 2002;73:395–9.
21. Burchiel KJ, Anderson VC, Favre J, Hammerstad JP. Comparison of pallidal and subthalamic nucleus deep brain stimulation for advanced Parkinson's disease: results of a randomized, blinded pilot study. Neurosurgery. 1999;45:1375–82.
22. Kumar R, Lozano AM, Montgomery E, Lang AE. Pallidotomy and deep brain stimulation of the pallidum and subthalamic nucleus in advanced Parkinson's disease. Mov Disord. 1998;13 Suppl 1:73–82.
23. Moruzzi G, Magoun HW. Brain stem reticular formation and activation of the EEG. Electroencephalogr Clin Neurophysiol. 1949;1:455–73.
24. Fuster JM. Effects of stimulation of brain stem on tachistoscopic perception. Science. 1958;127:150.
25. Kinomura S, Larsson J, Gulyas B, Roland PE. Activation by attention of the human reticular formation and thalamic intralaminar nuclei. Science. 1996;271:512–5.
26. Sturm V, Kuhner A, Schmitt HP, et al. Chronic electrical stimulation of the thalamic unspecific activating system in a patient with coma due to midbrain and upper brain stem infarction. Acta Neurochir (Wien). 1979;47:235–44.
27. Hassler R, Ore GD, Dieckmann G, et al. Behavioural and EEG arousal induced by stimulation of unspecific projection systems in a patient with post-traumatic apallic syndrome. Electroencephalogr Clin Neurophysiol. 1969;27:306.
28. McLardy T, Ervin F, Mark V, et al. Attempted inset-electrodes-arousal from traumatic coma: neuropathological findings. Trans Am Neurol Assoc. 1968;93:25–30.
29. Cohadon F. Deep brain stimulation in cases of prolonged traumatic unconsciousness. In: Lazorthes Y, Upton ARM, editors. Neurostimulation: an overview. New York: Futura Publishers; 1985.
30. Tsubokawa T, Yamamoto T, Katayama Y, et al. Deep-brain stimulation in a persistent vegetative state: follow-up results and criteria for selection of candidates. Brain Inj. 1990;4:315–27.
31. Katayama Y, Tsubokawa T, Yamamoto T, et al. Characterization and modification of brain activity with deep brain stimulation in patients in a persistent vegetative state: pain-related late positive component of cerebral evoked potential. Pacing Clin Electrophysiol. 1991;14:116–21.

32. Hosobuchi Y, Yingling C. The treatment of prolonged coma with neurostimulation. In: Devinsky O, Beric A, Dogali M, editors. Electrical and magnetic stimulation of the brain and spinal cord. New York: Raven; 1993. p. 247–52.
33. Giacino JT, Ashwal S, Childs N, et al. The minimally conscious state: definition and diagnostic criteria. Neurology. 2002;58:349–53.
34. Yamamoto T, Kobayashi K, Kasai M, et al. DBS therapy for the vegetative state and minimally conscious state. Acta Neurochir Suppl. 2005;93:101–4.
35. Adams JH, Graham DI, Jennett B. The neuropathology of the vegetative state after an acute brain insult. Brain. 2000;123(Pt 7):1327–38.
36. Schiff ND, Giacino JT, Kalmar K, et al. Behavioural improvements with thalamic stimulation after severe traumatic brain injury. Nature. 2007;448(7153):600–3.
37. Giacino JT, Kalmar K, Whyte J. The JFK Coma Recovery Scale-Revised: measurement characteristics and diagnostic utility. Arch Phys Med Rehabil. 2004;85:2020–9.
38. Lammi MH, Smith VH, Tate RL, Taylor CM. The minimally conscious state and recovery potential: a follow-up study 2 to 5 years after traumatic brain injury. Arch Phys Med Rehabil. 2005;86:746–54.
39. Laureys S, Berré J, Goldman S. Cerebral function in coma, vegetative state, minimally conscious state, locked-in syndrome and brain death. In: Vincent JL, editor. Yearbook of intensive care and emergency medicine. Berlin: Springer; 2001. p. 386–96.
40. Laureys S, Goldman S, Phillips C, et al. Impaired effective cortical connectivity in vegetative state: preliminary investigation using PET. Neuroimage. 1999;9:377–82.
41. Maxwell WL, MacKinnon MA, Smith DH, et al. Thalamic nuclei after human blunt head injury. J Neuropathol Exp Neurol. 2006;65:478–88.
42. Krout KE, Belzer RE, Loewy AD. Brainstem projections to midline and intralaminar thalamic nuclei of the rat. J Comp Neurol. 2002;448:53–101.
43. Schiff ND. Central thalamic deep-brain stimulation in the severely injured brain: rationale and proposed mechanisms of action. Ann N Y Acad Sci. 2009;1157:101–16.
44. Parvizi J, Damasio A. Consciousness and the brainstem. Cognition. 2001;79:135–60.
45. Fins JJ. Neuroethics and neuroimaging: moving toward transparency. Am J Bioeth. 2008;8(9):46–52.

Chapter 14
The Ethics of Managing Disorders of Consciousness

Athena Demertzi, Olivia Gosseries, Marie-Aurélie Bruno, Caroline Schnakers, Audrey Vanhaudenhuyse, Camille Chatelle, Vanessa Charland-Verville, Aurore Thibaut, Marie Thonnard, and Steven Laureys

Introduction

The introduction of the mechanical ventilator in the 1950s and the development of intensive care in the 1960s made it possible to sustain many patients' vegetative functions and allowed them to survive their severe injuries. Despite such advancement, in many cases, patients were found to suffer from altered states of consciousness, which had never been encountered before as these patients would normally die from apnea [1]. The imminent ethical impact of these profound states of unconsciousness was reflected in the composition of the first bioethical committees

---

A. Demertzi, M.Sc. (✉) • M.-A. Bruno, Ph.D. • C. Schnakers, Ph.D. • A. Vanhaudenhuyse, Ph.D. • C. Chatelle, M.Sc. • V. Charland-Verville, M.Sc. • A. Thibaut, M.Sc. • M. Thonnard, M.Sc. • S. Laureys, M.D., Ph.D.
Coma Science Group, Cyclotron Research Center, University of Liège,
Allée du 6 Août, Sart Tilman B30, 4000 Liège, Belgium

Department of Neurology, CHU University Hospital of Liège, Liège, Belgium
e-mail: a.demertzi@ulg.ac.be; ma.bruno@ulg.ac.be; c.schnakers@ulg.ac.be; avanhaudenhuyse@ulg.ac.be; camille.chatelle@ulg.ac.be; v.charland@student.ulg.ac.be; athibaut@student.ulg.ac.be; marie.thonnard@ulg.ac.be; steven.laureys@ulg.ac.be

O. Gosseries, M.Sc.
Coma Science Group, Cyclotron Research Center, University of Liège,
Allée du 6 Août, Sart Tilman B30, 4000 Liège, Belgium

Department of Neurology, CHU University Hospital of Liège, Liège, Belgium

National Fund for Scientific Research, Liège, Belgium
e-mail: ogosseries@ulg.ac.be

C. Schnakers, S. Laureys (eds.), *Coma and Disorders of Consciousness*,
DOI 10.1007/978-1-4471-2440-5_14, © Springer-Verlag London 2012

discussing the redefinition of life and the concept of therapeutic obstinacy. In 1968, the Ad Hoc Committee of Harvard Medical School published a milestone paper for the redefinition of death as irreversible coma and brain failure [2]. The committee mainly included several physicians, a theologian, a lawyer, and a historian of science, anticipating the medical, legal, and societal debates that were to follow. We will here give a brief overview of some ethical issues related to the concept of consciousness and the medical management of patients with disorders of consciousness (DOC) such as comatose, vegetative, and minimally conscious states that may be encountered in the intensive care setting. We will emphasize the problem of pain management and end-of-life decision-making.

Ethical Issues on Clinical Management

Confusions and controversies are often related to the way we define things. One such multifaceted term is consciousness, which has many divergent connotations [3]. The way we define consciousness is crucial, as it may govern our attitudes toward medical management of DOC. For example, in a wide survey ($n = 1,858$) among medical and paramedical professionals, we recently found that although the majority of healthcare workers denied the distinction between consciousness and the brain, more than one-third of medical and paramedical professionals still regarded mind and brain as separate entities. Such dualistic opinions may have implications to the formulation of scientific questions about the nature of consciousness, to clinical management of DOC, and to the reception of both by the general public [4]. We here adopt a perspective where consciousness is clinically defined as having two components, wakefulness and awareness [5]. Under this definition, many variant altered states of consciousness may be included. The most familiar of all is the transition from conscious wakefulness to deep sleep; the drowsier we become, the less aware we get of our surroundings and of ourselves. This implies that patients in coma and under anesthesia (i.e., pharmacological coma) are unaware because they cannot be awakened, even after noxious stimulation. The vegetative state (VS), now called unresponsive wakefulness syndrome (UWS), is defined as "wakefulness without awareness" where patients may open their eyes but never will exhibit nonreflex voluntary movements [6]. A patient in a minimally conscious state (MCS) may show some signs stating awareness (e.g., visual pursuit, orientation to pain, or nonsystematic command following) but is unable to communicate her or his thoughts or feelings [7]. Because these behavioral signs of consciousness often are small and fluctuating in time, this condition may be challenging to diagnose and differentiate from VS [8]. It has been suggested that once conscious awareness has been detected in a noncommunicative patient [9, 10], this may be a good reason to preserve life-sustaining aids [11]. However, the moral significance of preserved consciousness has been questioned on the grounds that it may not always be in patients' best interest to continue a severely disabled life [12].

One challenging issue is the conscious perception of pain in these patients. As defined by the Multi-Society Task Force on PVS, "pain and suffering refer to the unpleasant experiences that occur in response to stimulation of peripheral nociceptive receptors and their peripheral and central afferent pathways or that they may emanate endogenously from the depths of human self-perception" [13]. Thus, pain constitutes a conscious experience with a physical (nociception) and a psychological counterpart (suffering), suggesting that nociception by itself is not sufficient to cause suffering. The management of pain in patients with DOC is challenging because patients in VS/UWS or MCS cannot verbally or nonverbally communicate their feelings or experiences [1]. This is reflected on how clinicians perceive pain in these patients. According to recently surveyed attitudes among healthcare professionals, a majority of respondents supported that patients in MCS (96%) perceive pain whereas opinions were less clear for the patients in VS/UWS (56%) [14]. Considering these results on varying beliefs about pain perception in DOC, physicians and healthcare workers' views on analgesia and symptom management may also be affected. Since nearly half of the surveyed doctors expressed that VS/UWS patients do not feel pain, they could be expected to act accordingly, e.g., by not providing analgesic medication in these patients during care or during the dying process after withdrawal of artificial hydration and nutrition [15], the latter on the grounds that these patients may not experience suffering from hunger or thirst [16].

How are clinicians supposed to infer whether VS/UWS or MCS patients feel pain or suffering? At the patient's bedside, we are limited to evaluate the behavioral responsiveness to pain: if patients show no signs of voluntary movement (i.e., localizing the source of pain) in response to a noxious stimulus, it may be concluded they do not experience pain. Conscious but paralyzed "locked-in syndrome" patients, classically showing no movements or decerebrate (i.e., stereotyped extension)/ decorticate (i.e., stereotyped flexion) posturing, illustrate it is not necessarily the case. In response to noxious stimulation, DOC patients will frequently show increased arousal levels (evidenced by opening or widening of the eyes), increased respiratory/heart rate and blood pressure, or grimace-like/crying-like behavior. As all these responses are also seen in infants with anencephaly [17], they are considered to be of subcortical origin and not necessarily reflecting conscious perception of pain. However, the absence of one of these behavioral responses cannot be taken as a proof of the absence of conscious perception [18], and the inference of pain and suffering merely by observing behavioral responses may be misleading. Repeated clinical examinations performed by experienced examiners using standardized tools such as the recently proposed "Nociception Coma Scale" [19] are essential for the behavioral assessment of pain. Additional information coming from functional neuroimaging studies may help in the formulation of a clearer clinical picture. For example, in a positron emission tomography (PET) study, it was shown that VS/UWS patients may show cerebral processing of the noxious stimulus (activation of primary somatosensory areas) but the observed neural activity was isolated and disconnected from higher-order associative brain areas, which are considered necessary for conscious perception of pain [20]. It is important to stress that very different results were obtained in MCS patients where functional neuroimaging studies have shown a cerebral activation in a widespread cerebral network as compared to unresponsive patients, but similar to healthy controls, suggesting a potential pain perception in these patients [21]. In light of an incomplete pain perception in VS/UWS patients, the existing risk for misdiagnosis [8], the inconclusive drug-related effects in DOC [22] and the limitations of interpreting neuroimaging results [23], pain prophylaxis and drug treatment have been proposed for all patients suffering from DOC [24].

In intensive care settings, medical doctors and assisting staff are daily confronted with situations where clinical decisions are critical, such as continuing or withdrawing life-sustaining treatment. Treatment limitations can be different, depending on whether the decision is made preoperatively or after an intervention [25]. In the former case, it may come as a refusal of cardiopulmonary resuscitation (CPR) in case of cardiopulmonary arrest; in the latter case, it most usually comes as a decision to withdraw treatment such as the artificial respirator or artificial nutrition and hydration (ANH). CPR is almost automatically performed as an emergency therapy in order to restore heart beat and ceased breathing, unless the patient or the legal representative has refused it in advance as a do-not-resuscitate (DNR) order. Nevertheless, it should be noted that DNR orders do not necessarily prohibit other therapies; they rather authorize the physician to act on this specific therapy [26]. When the clinical condition of a patient has been stabilized and denoted as irreversible, decisions about ANH limitation may be considered. From a bioethical standpoint, withdrawing ANH is comparable to withdrawing mechanical ventilation, even if emotionally they may be perceived differently. In the ICU setting, the majority of deaths are the result of a medical decision to withhold or withdraw treatment [27]. Such decisions are evidence-based and rely on validated clinical or paraclinical markers of bad outcome [28]. Despite the controversy as to whether ANH constitutes a medical treatment [29], and thus should never be withdrawn from patients [30], most of the medical community (especially Anglo-Saxon) agrees on considering it as a medical therapy which can be refused by patients and surrogate decision makers [31]. Such decisions in the VS/UWS are only justified when a case is considered as irreversible [32]. Up to date, guidelines defining a definitive outcome in VS/UWS is that, if no recovery is observed within 3 months after a nontraumatic injury or 12 months after a traumatic injury, the condition of the patient can be considered as permanent [13].

The controversies around the clinical management at the end-of-life in DOC patients were reflected in a recent European survey ($n = 2{,}475$), where the majority of healthcare professionals (66%) agreed to withdraw treatment from chronic VS/UWS patients whereas only 28% agreed so for the chronic MCS; additionally, most clinicians wished not to be kept alive if they imagined themselves in a chronic VS (82%) and similar proportion (67%) agreed so if they imagined themselves in a chronic MCS [33]. Geographical region and religion were among the factors that explained most of the variance in the responses [33]. The detected differences between the two states could be due to the existing legal ambiguity around MCS, which may have influenced the surveyed participants to differentiate between expressing preferences for self versus others, by implicitly recognizing that the latter could be a step on the slippery slope to euthanasia.

Clinicians' opinions appear much more uniform with regard to brain death [34]. As mentioned earlier, the Ad Hoc Committee of the Harvard Medical School went on to redefine death as a consequence of the technological advancements in the intensive care, where patients could sustain their severe injuries but maintain the function of vital organs [2]. It was, hence, possible to dissociate between cardiac, respiratory, and brain functions, which in turn required an alternative definition of death, moving from a cardiorespiratory toward a neurocentric formulation (i.e., irreversible coma). According to the latter, death can be viewed either as death of the whole brain or of the brainstem [35] or as neocortical [36]. The first two are defined as the irreversible cessation of the organism as a whole, differing in their anatomical interpretation [37], whereas the last solely requires the irreversible loss of the capacity of consciousness and social interaction but has never convinced medical or legal scholars. The main utility of the introduction of brain death is that it permitted vital organ procurement for transplantation with the application of ethical restrictions, such as the dead donor rule (i.e., a patient has to be declared dead before the removal of life-sustaining organs). Based on the neocortical definition of death, however, both VS/UWS and MCS patients can be declared dead. It has been argued that the neocortical definition is conceptually inadequate and practically unfeasible, especially in lack of a complete understanding of higher-order conscious functioning; hence, DOC patients are not dead [27] and organ donation options in these patients should be excluded since they violate the dead donor rule [38]—despite opposing opinions to abandon this ethical axiom [39].

Legal Issues in Disorders of Consciousness

Managing patients with disorders of consciousness may require the mediation of legal authorities in order to regulate ambiguous and controversial issues, such as end-of-life decisions. When end-of-life wishes have not been earlier formulated as an advance directive (i.e., written statement completed by a competent person in anticipation of her/his future incompetence, expressing personal treatment preferences and formal surrogacy appointment), then a surrogate decision maker is eligible to take responsibility of the patient's clinical management. The way the legal representative should act on behalf of the patient is a progressive one. The surrogate should first attempt to follow the wishes of the patient as closely as possible the way they were expressed before the accident, either orally or as advance directives. When the wishes are unknown and an advance directive is not available, the surrogate decision maker should try to reproduce the patients' preferences based on their history and personal values. When this is not possible the decisions should rely on more objective markers that determine the patients' best interest (e.g. likelihood of recovery, pain management, impact on family) [25, 40]. The proxy decision maker should mediate trying to maximize patients' self-determination and protect their interests on the principles of beneficence and nonmaleficence (i.e., ongoing treatment may be judged to be futile on the basis of low likelihood of significant recovery) [41].

The use of advance directives could also be considered as a means to regulate cost savings in the end-of-life; once the wishes of a terminal patient are known, care can be taken as to constrain extraordinary means and spare the available resources on other urgent cases. However, no such rationale corresponds to reality, and advance directives, together with hospice care and the elimination of futile care, have not contributed to the effective regulation of the economics of dying [42]. Treatment resources are not unlimited and despite care for a good death sometimes physicians need to do with the means they have available. The allocation of resources and the economics at the end-of-life have not yet been fully determined for DOC patients. In ICU medicine some unwritten rules can facilitate decisions as to who is to be treated, like the "first come" principle or "who will most likely benefit from the intensive care" [43]. However, for chronic DOC cases, information on resource allocation is often lacking. This may be due to the nature of chronic VS/UWS and MCS patients. These are severely brain-damaged patients for whom the dilemma on treating becomes crucial either because treatments are not guaranteed as successful (i.e., the condition is too bad to be treated) or unkind (i.e., the quality of life of those surviving is not acceptable) which may lead to an unwise way to allocate the available resources [43].

The legal provisions concerning the end-of-life issues in DOC differ from country to country. In the United States, where a patient-centered medical framework has been adopted, the patient is allowed to participate in the regulation of her/his own medical care. In the case of DOC, legal representatives in close collaboration with the clinical staff and in line with the patients' previously expressed wishes may decide together about the long-term care of irreversibly comatose patients. There are times, however, when conflicts of interests arise while making such decisions either between family and physicians, such as in the Quinlan case [44], or among family members, like the more recent Schiavo case [45]. As most often such cases require the mediation of the court, they may have a wider publicity where the public opinion can come into play and may lead to societal movements on pro-life versus right-to-die action groups [46]. In Europe, there are more subtle differences in the way treatment limitation is perceived, especially between Northern (more right-to-die oriented) and Southern European countries (more pro-life oriented) [33]. In general, decisions for treatment limitation (usually concerning ANH) need to be taken after reference to the court. Exceptions are the Netherlands, Belgium, Switzerland, and Scandinavian countries where no court mediation is needed for limiting treatment in DOC patients [47].

Conclusions

The ethical issues, accrued from the study and management of DOC patients, are variant and multifaceted. The medical, legal, and public controversies are partly shaped by how different people think about these issues and in many cases are country-dependent. It is, hence, necessary that a uniform ethical framework has to be shaped to guide clinicians and caregivers in terms of clinical outcome, prognosis, and medical management.

References

1. Laureys S, Boly M. What is it like to be vegetative or minimally conscious? Curr Opin Neurol. 2007;20:609–13.
2. Report of the Ad Hoc Committee of the Harvard Medical School to Examine the Definition of Brain Death. A definition of irreversible coma. JAMA. 1968;205:337–40.
3. Zeman A. Consciousness. Brain. 2001;124:1263–89.
4. Demertzi A, Liew C, Ledoux D, et al. Dualism persists in the science of mind. Ann N Y Acad Sci. 2009;1157:1–9.
5. Posner J, Saper C, Schiff N, Plum F, editors. Plum and Posner's diagnosis of stupor and coma. 4th ed. New York: Oxford University Press; 2007.
6. Jennett B, Plum F. Persistent vegetative state after brain damage. A syndrome in search of a name. Lancet. 1972;1:734–7.
7. Giacino JT, Ashwal S, Childs N, et al. The minimally conscious state: definition and diagnostic criteria. Neurology. 2002;58:349–53.
8. Schnakers C, Vanhaudenhuyse A, Giacino JT, et al. Diagnostic accuracy of the vegetative and minimally conscious state: clinical consensus versus standardized neurobehavioral assessment. BMC Neurol. 2009;9:35.
9. Owen AM, Coleman MR, Boly M, Davis MH, Laureys S, Pickard JD. Detecting awareness in the vegetative state. Science. 2006;313:1402.
10. Monti MM, Vanhaudenhuyse A, Coleman MR, et al. Willful modulation of brain activity in disorders of consciousness. N Engl J Med. 2010;362:579–89.
11. Horne M (2009) Are people in a persistent vegetative state conscious? Monash Bioeth Rev. 28:12–1–12.
12. Kahane G, Savulescu J. Brain damage and the moral significance of consciousness. J Med Philos. 2009;34:6–26.
13. International Association for the Study of Pain. Classification of chronic pain: descriptions of chronic pain syndromes and definitions of pain terms, Task force on taxonomy. Seatle: IASP Press; 1994.
14. Demertzi A, Schnakers C, Ledoux D, et al. Different beliefs about pain perception in the vegetative and minimally conscious states: a European survey of medical and paramedical professionals. Prog Brain Res. 2009;177:329–38.
15. Fins JJ. Affirming the right to care, preserving the right to die: disorders of consciousness and neuroethics after Schiavo. Palliat Support Care. 2006;4:169–78.
16. Ahronheim JC, Gasner MR. The sloganism of starvation. Lancet. 1990;335:278–9.
17. The Medical Task Force on Anencephaly. The infant with anencephaly. N Engl J Med. 1990;322:669–74.
18. McQuillen MP. Can people who are unconscious or in the "vegetative state" perceive pain? Issues Law Med. 1991;6:373–83.
19. Schnakers C, Chatelle C, Vanhaudenhuyse A, et al. The Nociception Coma Scale: a new tool to assess nociception in disorders of consciousness. Pain. 2010;148:215–9.
20. Laureys S, Faymonville ME, Peigneux P, et al. Cortical processing of noxious somatosensory stimuli in the persistent vegetative state. Neuroimage. 2002;17:732–41.
21. Boly M, Faymonville ME, Schnakers C, et al. Perception of pain in the minimally conscious state with PET activation: an observational study. Lancet Neurol. 2008;7:1013–20.
22. Demertzi A, Vanhaudenhuyse A, Bruno MA, et al. Is there anybody in there? Detecting awareness in disorders of consciousness. Expert Rev Neurother. 2008;8:1719–30.

23. Poldrack RA. The role of fMRI in cognitive neuroscience: where do we stand? Curr Opin Neurobiol. 2008;18:223–7.
24. Schnakers C, Zasler ND. Pain assessment and management in disorders of consciousness. Curr Opin Neurol. 2007;20:620–6.
25. Bernat JL. Ethical issues in the perioperative management of neurologic patients. Neurol Clin. 2004;22:457–71.
26. Youngner SJ. Do-not-resuscitate orders: no longer secret, but still a problem. Hastings Cent Rep. 1987;17:24–33.
27. Laureys S. Science and society: death, unconsciousness and the brain. Nat Rev Neurosci. 2005;6:899–909.
28. Boveroux P, Kirsch M, Boly M, et al. Évaluation du pronostic neurologique dans les encéphalopathies postanoxiques. Réanimation. 2008;17:613–7.
29. Bernat JL, Beresford HR. The controversy over artificial hydration and nutrition. Neurology. 2006;66:1618–9.
30. Rosner F. Why nutrition and hydration should not be withheld from patients. Chest. 1993;104:1892–6.
31. Steinbrook R, Lo B. Artificial feeding–solid ground, not a slippery slope. N Engl J Med. 1988;318:286–90.
32. Royal College of Physicians. The vegetative state: guidance on diagnosis and management. Clin Med. 2003;3:249–54.
33. Demertzi A, Ledoux D, Bruno MA, et al. Attitudes towards end-of-life issues in disorders of consciousness: a European survey. J Neurol. 2011;258(6):1058–65.
34. Bernat JL, Steven L. The concept and practice of brain death. Prog Brain Res. 2005;150:369–79.
35. Bernat JL. Ethical issues in neurology. 2nd ed. Boston: Butterworth Heinemann; 2002.
36. Brierley JB, Graham DI, Adams JH, Simpsom JA. Neocortical death after cardiac arrest. A clinical, neurophysiological, and neuropathological report of two cases. Lancet. 1971;2:560–5.
37. Bernat JL. A defense of the whole-brain concept of death. Hastings Cent Rep. 1998;28:14–23.
38. Engelhardt K. Organ donation and permanent vegetative state. Lancet. 1998;351:211.
39. Truog RD, Robinson WM. Role of brain death and the dead-donor rule in the ethics of organ transplantation. Crit Care Med. 2003;31:2391–6.
40. Bernat JL. Clinical ethics and the Law. In: Bernat JL, editor. Ethical issues in neurology. Boston: Butterworth Heinemann; 2002. p. 79–107.
41. Bernat JL. The persistent vegetative state and related states. In: Bernat JL, editor. Ethical issues in neurology. Boston: Butterworth Heinemann; 2002. p. 283–305.
42. Emanuel EJ, Emanuel LL. The economics of dying. The illusion of cost savings at the end of life. N Engl J Med. 1994;330:540–4.
43. Jennett B. Editorial: resource allocation for the severely brain damaged. Arch Neurol. 1976;33:595–7.
44. Beresford HR. The Quinlan decision: problems and legislative alternatives. Ann Neurol. 1977;2:74–81.
45. Quill TE. Terri Schiavo –a tragedy compounded. N Engl J Med. 2005;352:1630–3.
46. Wijdicks EFM. Law and bioethics. In: Wijdicks EFM, editor. The comatose patient. New York: Oxford University Press; 2008. p. 201–16.
47. Jennett B. Ethical issues. In: Jennett B, editor. The vegetative state: medical facts, ethical and legal dilemmas. Cambridge: Cambridge University Press; 2002. p. 97–125.

Chapter 15
Future Perspectives of Clinical Coma Science

Steven Laureys and Caroline Schnakers

Redefining Disorders of Consciousness

As illustrated in the previous chapters, the clinical management of disorders of consciousness remains very difficult, but technological advances in neuroimaging and in EEG-based brain–computer interfaces are now offering new ways to improve the diagnostic, prognostic, and therapeutic management of these challenging conditions. We believe the recent international clinical research efforts in this challenging field are heralding a new era of consciousness science and coma management [1].

Following severe brain damage and coma, some patients may awaken (i.e., open the eyes) but remain unresponsive (i.e., only showing reflex movements). In Europe, this clinical syndrome was initially termed apallic syndrome and coma vigil; but it was later redefined as vegetative state (VS). Since its description more than 35 years ago, an increasing number of functional neuroimaging and event related potential studies [2] have shown that it sometimes may be difficult to make strong claims about *vegetative* patients' awareness [3]. This situation is further complicated when patients have underlying deficits in verbal or nonverbal communication functions, such as aphasia, agnosia, or apraxia [4].

S. Laureys, M.D., Ph.D. (✉)
Coma Science Group, Cyclotron Research Center, University of Liège,
Allée du 6 Août, Sart Tilman B30, 4000 Liège, Belgium

Department of Neurology, University Hospital of Liège,
Liège, Belgium
e-mail: steven.laureys@ulg.ac.be

C. Schnakers, Ph.D.
Coma Science Group, Cyclotron Research Center, University of Liège,
Allée du 6 Août, Sart Tilman B30, 4000 Liège, Belgium
e-mail: c.schnakers@ulg.ac.be

C. Schnakers, S. Laureys (eds.), *Coma and Disorders of Consciousness*,
DOI 10.1007/978-1-4471-2440-5_15, © Springer-Verlag London 2012

It appears that part of the healthcare, media, and lay public continue to feel some unease regarding the unintended denigrating *vegetable-like* connotation seemingly intrinsic to the term VS. The European Task Force on Disorders of Consciousness, therefore, recently proposed an alternative name: *unresponsive wakefulness syndrome* (UWS) [5]. Hence, physicians are recently offered to refer to these patients as UWS, a more neutral and descriptive term, pertaining to patients showing a number of clinical signs (hence syndrome) of unresponsiveness (i.e., without response to commands or oriented voluntary movements) in the presence of wakefulness (i.e., eye opening). In contrast to coma, which is an acute condition lasting no more than some days or weeks; VS/UWS can be a chronic condition lasting years or remain permanent.

Those patients who do recover, classically evolve to a minimally conscious state, defined by the presence of nonreflex voluntary movements such as orientation to pain, eye tracking, or reproducible albeit inconsistent command following. By definition, MCS patients cannot communicate their thoughts or wishes [6]. Finally, in pseudocoma or locked-in syndrome (LIS), patients may awaken from coma fully conscious but paralyzed, only able to communicate by eye movements. The medical and ethical management of these vulnerable patients is very complex and a recent paper reviewed the even more challenging (but fortunately very rare) situation of LIS in children [7]. Locked-in patients illustrate how difficult it can be to make inferences about subjective conscious awareness in severely motor impaired.

A Brief History of Coma

Historically, the seat of consciousness was widely believed to be in the heart, and the absence of heartbeat was regarded as the clinical sign of death. Neurological scientific evidence has superseded such thinking and shown that consciousness, an emergent property of neural activity, resides in the brain [1]. Since the invention of the positive-pressure mechanical respirator, it has become possible to truly dissociate cardiac, respiratory, and brain functions in individuals who are in a coma. Patients who would previously have died from apnea are now able to survive in profound comatose states that had never been encountered before. This technological progress forced modern medicine to redefine the diagnosis of death and move from its ancient cardiorespiratory-centered definition to a neurocentric one, where death is defined as the irreversible loss of all brainstem reflexes (including the breathing reflex). Since the introduction of this clinical definition, not a single patient who was declared brain dead has ever regained consciousness.

The origin of coma research, as a science, probably dates to 1966 when Fred Plum and Jerome Posner published the first edition of their classic text *The Diagnosis of Stupor and Coma* [8]. For the first time, researchers correlated clinical findings that were derived from the examination of patients in comatose states with pathological findings, and proposed a pathophysiology of consciousness. In 1974, Bryan Jennett and colleagues published the Glasgow Coma Scale [9] and, in the next year, the Glasgow Outcome Scale [10]. These standardized scoring systems enabled the performance of multicenter clinical trials and epidemiological studies that resulted in the development of rational algorithms for the treatment (or withdrawal thereof) of comatose patients.

Pioneers such as Jennett and Plum revolutionized the field of acute brain injury. However, the excitement of the 1970s was followed by a return to therapeutic nihilism (i.e., the assumption that patients with chronic disorders of consciousness are uniformly hopeless cases) and a marked decrease of scientific interest in disorders of consciousness. Coma research nearly got comatose. Only recently, partly incited by advances in the field of functional neuroimaging, did the study of coma and related states undergo a revival [11].

New Ways of Showing Signs of Consciousness

The clinical studies conducted, since the 1970s, have illustrated how challenging it is to disentangle reflex behavior from voluntary behavior—a problem that can potentially lead to diagnostic error. We are confined to inferring the presence of awareness from a patient's motor responsiveness. The differential diagnosis of disorders of consciousness, hence, may be challenging. The rate of misdiagnosis is approximately 40%, and new methods are required to complement bedside testing, particularly if the patient's capacity to show behavioral signs of awareness is diminished [12].

Functional neuroimaging now offers the possibility to directly measure the brain's activity, not only at rest or during passive stimulation, but also in response to commands [11]. Assessing resting state brain metabolism using fluorodeoxyglucose PET, a recent study could disentangle vegetative from locked-in patients by an automatic procedure based on machine learning [13]. A sparse probabilistic Bayesian learning framework called "relevance vector machine" correctly classified all included scans as conscious (i.e., locked-in) or unconscious (i.e., vegetative/unresponsive). Such automated user-independent, classification tools of cerebral metabolic images obtained in coma survivors could become a useful tool for the automated PET-based diagnosis of altered states of consciousness.

In the same line, resting state functional MRI study can now quantify the integrity of the brain's connectivity pattern in the so-called *default mode network* in pathological alterations of consciousness [14]. The default network is defined as a set of areas, encompassing posterior-cingulate/precuneus, anterior-cingulate/mesiofrontal cortex, and temporoparietal junctions, which show more activity at rest than during attention-demanding tasks. Connectivity was investigated using probabilistic independent component analysis, and an automated template-matching component selection approach. Connectivity in all default network areas was found to be negatively correlated with the degree of clinical consciousness impairment, ranging from healthy controls and locked-in syndrome to minimally conscious, vegetative, then coma patients. Furthermore, precuneus connectivity was found to be significantly stronger in minimally conscious patients as compared with unconscious patients; and locked-in syndrome patient's default network connectivity was not significantly different from controls. Prospective studies in a larger patient population are needed in order to evaluate the prognostic value of the presented methodology.

Communicating via a Scanner

fMRI activation studies classically measure the brain's response to external sensory stimuli. For example, Qin et al. [15] have studied auditory processing in 11 DOC patients using an auto-referential attention-grabbing stimulus, the patient's own name. They reported a linear correlation between activation of the limbic system (anterior cingulate cortex) and the level of consciousness as quantified by coma recovery scores. However, such *passive* stimulation induced by brain activation does permit to make strong claims about the patient's consciousness.

Now, Monti and Vanhaudenhuyse et al. [16] have been using a so-called *active* paradigm where patients are instructed to follow simple commands. Their study enrolled 54 DOC cases of different etiology in imaging centers in Cambridge and Liège, asking patients to perform two mental imagery tasks: *imagine playing tennis* (activating motor areas) and *imagine walking around in your house* (activating parahippocampal brain regions). Of the 31 patients previously diagnosed as MCS, only one was able to show reliable fMRI activation in the expected brain areas, illustrating that the employed technique only has a sensitivity of 3% in minimally conscious DOC patients (i.e., has a 97% false negative rate). It is more difficult to calculate the sensitivity and specificity of the technique in VS/UWS patients given that we do not have a *gold standard* of consciousness. Indeed, in the published case series, 4 out of 23 clinically unconscious patients showed fMRI signs of command following and hence of consciousness (i.e., 17%); but given the known low sensitivity, it could be that other patients might have been (minimally) conscious yet were unable to do the task or show statistically significant brain activation. However, in those individual patients where reliable and long-lasting (>30 s) command-related fMRI activation was observed, there seems no logical alternative explanation other than that they repeatedly understood and replied to the commands and hence truly showed conscious awareness [17].

In addition to show proof of consciousness, fMRI is being used to communicate with some (very exceptional) DOC patients. Indeed, one clinically noncommunicative patient studied in the Liège University Hospital was shown to correctly answer five out of six simple questions regarding his family members' names [16]. Here, it was set that to communicate "*yes*," one should imagine playing tennis (and hence motor area activation was identified using an automated user-independent relative-similarity classifier) and to communicate "*no*," the spatial navigation task should be performed (activating parahippocampal areas). fMRI muscle-independent communication currently even goes beyond such yes–no answers to closed questions and is offering the possibility to answer multiple choice questions [18]. Evidently, these data should be seen as proofs of concept rather than as a practical means to truly assure long-term communication. EEG based communication devices, called brain–computer interfaces, are, therefore, being developed as a more practical, transportable, and cheaper alternative.

Similarly, to the described fMRI *active* paradigms, EEG-based technology will aim to answer two questions—*Is the patient conscious?* and, if the answer is affirmative, *What is that consciousness like?*—needing functional communication. The practical utility of demonstrating voluntary brain activity using nonclinical means has already been translated to clinical use—illustrated in the case of a 21-year old comatose woman who failed to show any motor sign of conscious awareness up to 49 days after an extensive brainstem and thalamic stroke [19]. Only EEG evoked-potential based command following (i.e., counting a target name in a list of names), shown at the intensive care unit, permitted to make the diagnosis of complete locked-in syndrome. Future multicentric trials are awaited to validate the possible prognostic value of these tests.

Predicting and Improving the Outcome

In many patients with disorders of consciousness, it remains difficult to reliably predict the chances of functional recovery. However, MRI techniques such as spectroscopy and diffusion tensor imaging are improving our possibilities to quantify the neuronal damage. Magnetic resonance spectroscopy now permits to reveal axonal sprouting in exceptional cases of late recovery [20]. Such demonstration of axonal sprouting after sometimes very long time intervals of several years disproves the old dogma that neural plasticity is limited to the acute or subacute phase of head trauma.

Finally, the widespread therapeutic nihilism with regards to chronic disorders of consciousness is being challenged by new evidence derived from the use of deep-brain stimulation. Posttraumatic minimally conscious state patients are undergoing bilateral thalamic stimulation, improving cognitive function and resulted in a return to functional object use and intelligible verbalization [21]. The usefulness of deep brain stimulation in this setting again awaits confirmation from studies that include larger cohorts of patients, but the evidence to date indicates that the technique can offer a real therapeutic option in well-chosen patients (selected on the basis of functional neuroimaging results).

In the recovery from coma, the acquisition of interactive verbal or nonverbal communication represents an important milestone—the ability to communicate their wishes concerning treatment options allows these vulnerable patients to exert their right to autonomy. Rapid advances in the development of brain–computer interfaces mean that clinically noncommunicative coma survivors can finally have a voice of their own [22]. We predict that real-time functional MRI and EEG-mediated technology will offer these patients nonmuscle-dependent channels of communication, enabling them to express their thoughts, control their environment, and increase their quality-of-life.

Changing the Spectrum of Coma

Clearly, it is a thrilling time for the field of acute-brain injury. The gray zones between the different disorders of consciousness in the clinical spectrum following coma are beginning to be better defined by the addition of powerful imaging methodology to bedside clinical assessment. We foresee that in a yet-to-be-discovered fraction of patients who are currently considered to be vegetative, electromyography, event-related potential, and functional MRI techniques will reveal signs of consciousness that are unattainable by bedside clinical assessment. These novel technological means will change the existing behaviorally defined boundaries between the various consciousness disorders (Fig. 15.1). In a next step, these high-tech devices will permit some of these clinically *noncommunicative* patients to correspond their thoughts and wishes via nonmotor pathways. However, it should be

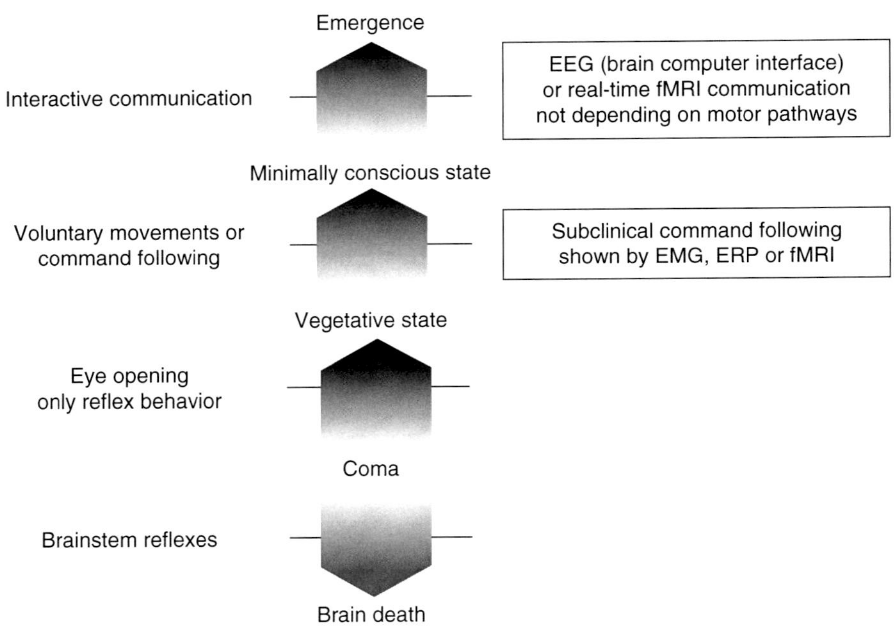

Fig. 15.1 Patients in a coma may become brain dead (when brainstem reflexes are irreversibly lost) or progress to a vegetative state (clinically defined as wakefulness solely accompanied by reflex behavior); next patients may transition to a minimally conscious state (i.e., the patient shows signs of command following or other nonreflexive movements); the restoration of interactive communication indicates the emergence from this stage in the clinical spectrum of recovery from coma. Novel technological means are changing these behaviorally defined boundaries. In the future, electromyography (*EMG*), event-related potential (*ERP*) and functional MRI (*fMRI*) techniques might reveal signs of consciousness that are unattainable by bedside clinical assessment in a yet-to-be-discovered fraction of patients who are currently considered to be vegetative. In a next step, these high-tech devices might permit some of these patients to communicate their thoughts and wishes via nonmotor pathways

stressed that these exciting developments are not yet reality. The first hurdle to be overcome before the methodologies discussed above can enter clinical practice relates to ethical concerns. We side with a proposed ethical framework that emphasizes the need to achieve a balance between the protection of patients with disorders of consciousness and the ability to perform research that can lead to medical progress [23]. Most of the advances in coma science discussed above are based on single-case studies. Only large-scale multicenter clinical trials will enable these research tools to find their way into evidence-based care that really influences the lives of individuals with a disorder of consciousness.

References

1. Laureys S, Boly M. The changing spectrum of coma. Nat Clin Pract Neurol. 2008; 4(10):544–6.
2. Bruno MA, Gosseries O, Ledoux D, et al. Assessment of consciousness with electrophysiological and neurological imaging techniques. Curr Opin Crit Care. 2011;17(2):146–51.
3. Monti MM, Laureys S, Owen AM. The vegetative state. Brit Med J. 2010;341:3765.
4. Majerus S, Bruno MA, Schnakers C, et al. The problem of aphasia in the assessment of consciousness in brain-damaged patients. Prog Brain Res. 2009;177:49–61.
5. European Task Force on Disorders of Consciousness. Unresponsive wakefulness syndrome: a new name for the vegetative state or apallic syndrome. BMC Med. 2010;1(8):68.
6. Giacino JT, Schnakers C, Rodriguez-Moreno D, et al. Behavioral assessment in patients with disorders of consciousness: gold standard or fool's gold? Prog Brain Res. 2009;177:33–48.
7. Bruno MA, Schnakers C, Damas F, et al. Locked-in syndrome in children: report of five cases and review of the literature. Pediatr Neurol. 2010;41(4):237–46.
8. Plum F, Posner JB. The diagnosis of stupor and coma. 1st ed. Philadelphia: Davis, F.A; 1966.
9. Teasdale G, Jennett B. Assessment of coma and impaired consciousness. A practical scale. Lancet. 1974;2(7872):81–4.
10. Jennett B, Bond M. Assessment of outcome after severe brain damage. Lancet. 1975;1(7905):480–4.
11. Owen A, Coleman M, Boly M, et al. Detecting awareness in the vegetative state. Science. 2006;313(5792):1402.
12. Schnakers C, Vanhaudenhuyse A, Giacino J, et al. Diagnostic accuracy of the vegetative and minimally conscious state: clinical consensus versus standardized neurobehavioral assessment. BMC Neurol. 2009;9:35.
13. Phillips CL, Bruno MA, Maquet P, et al. "Relevance vector machine" consciousness classifier applied to cerebral metabolism of vegetative and locked-in patients. Neuroimage. 2011;56(2):797–808.
14. Vanhaudenhuyse A, Demertzi A, Schabus M, et al. Two distinct neuronal networks mediate the awareness of environment and of self. J Cogn Neurosci. 2011;23(3):570–8.
15. Qin P, Di H, Liu Y, et al. Anterior cingulate activity and the self in disorders of consciousness. Hum Brain Mapp. 2010;31(12):1993–2002.
16. Monti MM, Vanhaudenhuyse A, Coleman MR, et al. Willful modulation of brain activity in disorders of consciousness. N Engl J Med. 2010;62(7):579–89.
17. Stins JF, Laureys S. Thought translation, tennis and Turing tests in the vegetative state. Phenom Cogn Sci. 2009;8:361–70.
18. Sorger B, Dahmen B, Reithler J, et al. Another kind of 'BOLD Response': answering multiple-choice questions via online decoded single-trial brain signals. Prog Brain Res. 2009;177:275–92.

19. Schnakers C, Perrin F, Schabus M, et al. Detecting consciousness in a total locked-in syndrome: an active event-related paradigm. Neurocase. 2009;15(4):271–7.
20. Voss HU, Uluc AM, Dyke JP, et al. Possible axonal regrowth in late recovery from the minimally conscious state. J Clin Invest. 2006;116(7):2005–11.
21. Schiff ND, Fins JJ. Deep brain stimulation and cognition: moving from animal to patient. Curr Opin Neurol. 2007;20(6):638–42.
22. Kubler A, Furdea A, Halder S, et al. A brain-computer interface controlled auditory event-related potential (p300) spelling system for locked-in patients. Ann N Y Acad Sci. 2009;1157:90–100.
23. Fins JJ, Schiff ND, Foley KM. Late recovery from the minimally conscious state: ethical and policy implications. Neurology. 2007;68(4):304–7.

Index

C. Schnakers, S. Laureys (eds.), *Coma and Disorders of Consciousness*,
DOI 10.1007/978-1-4471-2440-5,

FSC
www.fsc.org
MIX
Papier | Fördert
gute Waldnutzung
FSC® C083411

Kolibri 360 GmbH
Ferdinand-Jühlke-Straße 7
99095 Erfurt, Deutschland
produktsicherheit@kolibri360.de